Awkward Bitch

My Life With MS

Marlo Donato Parmelee

authorHOUSE®

AuthorHouse™ UK Ltd.
500 Avebury Boulevard
Central Milton Keynes, MK9 2BE
www.authorhouse.co.uk
Phone: 08001974150

First published by AuthorHouse 6/23/2009

ISBN: 978-1-4389-9048-4 (sc)

This book is printed on acid-free paper.

Cover illustration by Anthony War

In Loving Memory of Harriet Kearns

Acknowledgements

Thank you to:

my twin flame William, for your unwavering love,
support, strength, and encouragement. You make
me want to be a better person.
my mom Kathleen Donato, for always believing
in me. You are a bright light in this world and the
brightest light in my life.
my dad Mario R. Donato, for being a guiding star.
It's been 10 years since your death and you still
hold my hand.
my sisters Lisa, Lorraine, and Colleen. The three
of you have loved and encouraged me since day
one. Thanks for your faith in me.
my content editor Siobhan Curham, for your
incredible guidance and encouragement.
my Aunt Harriet, a kindred fighting soul,
for believing in this book from the moment I
mentioned the idea.

my best friend Laura, who has known I was a bitch
before I was the awkward one, and still loves me. I
love you too.

my *Petit Prince* Colin, for your friendship,
support, and life-saving humour. I can't imagine
life without you.

my friend and cover artist Anthony War, for
capturing the spirit of the book just how I
imagined it.

my friends and extended family members, for your
tolerance of me and belief in my capabilities

my outstanding doctors and nurses, especially
Professor Gavin Giovannoni, whom I feel fortunate
and privileged to be in the care of.

my unlikely muses, Peter Jackson and Alan Lee,
whose inspiring interviews regarding *The Lord of
the Rings*, was listened to during the writing of
this entire book (no joke).

Prologue

இ

It's 10 a.m. on Monday, the 23rd of July, 2007, and I am sitting alone in a waiting room in one of the oldest hospitals in London. The room is a dull shade of I don't know what. Despite my in-depth knowledge of colour, I can't really say what the shade is. The ceiling is showing its age with evidence of leaks from maybe 100 years ago. I wonder how many people have sat in this room before me. Thoughts are racing through my head like *I don't think I can go through with this*.

My bladder is full beyond capacity and I know that any minute I am going to piss myself. A fish tank that I foolishly chose to sit next to taunts me. Observing its filter bubble and make swishing noises has now become unbearable. Coupled with the fish tank water torture is a sign on the wall that reads 'Toilet' with an arrow pointing down a short hallway.

The toilet is so close, only behind the wall to my right. My palms are sweating as I glance down at the empty litre water bottle I am clenching between my hands. I frantically look around for the doctor and manage to catch the nurse's attention instead.

'Excuse me,' I mutter in a barely audible voice that doesn't even sound like mine. 'Excuse me, I....'

The nurse looks like she is coming over to me, but then gets distracted by a patient being wheeled through the door. She takes her eyes off me and directs all her attention to this new patient.

How the hell did I end up here? I think. *What must I look like?* I check my reflection in the fish tank. I go through a mental checklist: hair in place, check; mascara on, check; red lipstick perfect, check; bladder bursting, fuck it.

At that moment I make a split decision, typical of me in my life. I rise from my chair and race to the toilet as fast as my Gucci heels and awkward gait will carry me. What a relief this pee is! It is like no other! I return to my seat feeling a sense of great satisfaction and then guilt.

You see, I am not allowed to pee today; not yet. I am here for an ultrasound scan of my bladder and kidneys. I am supposed to drink my bottle of water, hold my pee, and wait for the doctor to come get me, take me in the dark scanning room, and scan my bladder.

After the scan, I am supposed to pee and then go back in the room for another scan of my bladder. The point is to see how it empties; making sure no residual urine gets left behind.

But now I've gone and ruined everything. The doctor will be here any moment and I will have to tell him what I did. I start laughing to myself. All the other patients seem to be holding their bladders just fine, and most of them are double my age or more!

Dr. Hogarth comes out and says, 'OK, Marlo, are you ready?'

'I've been a bad patient,' I answer, looking deep into his eyes for forgiveness.

He knows straight away. 'You peed?'

'Yes,' I admit. It is like admitting a crime to a police officer. 'I had to do it,' I said. 'I was ready to go in my pants.'

'OK,' he says compassionately. 'Drink more water and I'll come back for you in twenty minutes.'

'That's sounds good or even fifteen minutes will do,' I say and watch him walk away. As my bladder starts to quickly fill up again, I begin daydreaming, anything to get away from my present situation.

I start thinking of a time when I used to work in New York. On one particular day, I was running up Fifth Avenue with a Starbucks

Caramel Macchiato in one hand, a Chanel handbag in the other, wearing giant Jackie-O sunglasses, when a Japanese lady stopped me to pose for *JJ* magazine.

'Your look is cute!' she said. 'We take picture of you for Japanese magazine?' she asked, pointing me in the direction of a Japanese man with a long-lensed camera. '*Hai,*' I said, utilising some of the Japanese I learned from years working for Chanel on 57th Street. 'But I only have *choto mate* (one moment),' I told her, and posed for the photographer while she directed me how to stand. A group of tourists formed a circle around me to see what was going on.

I laugh to myself and look back into the fish tank. I don't look like that girl photographed in *JJ* magazine anymore. I don't look worse. Some might argue I look better. My husband would probably think so. I might be inclined to think so too, except for the polka-dot marks now covering so many parts of my body. Those are from the 335 times I have stuck a needle in myself in the past two years.

I sigh. No, I don't look like her. I *can't* look like her. Not after all that's happened. Not after crawling out of a tube station thinking I was dying. Not after all the times bending on the floor to pin famous people's trousers whilst going blind in one eye. Not after stumbling all over London, Paris, Miami, and New York in one week. Not after my band playing Trafalgar Square: THE Trafalgar Square! Not after being on public radio and television in one year. Not after my diagnosis.

No, I am not that girl, I think to myself. I look again into the fish tank and smile at my reflection. *I am better than that girl. I am better.* My thoughts are interrupted by Dr. Hogarth, who signals that he will get me in a minute. That is encouraging because I have now had three cups of water from the waiting room cooler and my bladder is reaching bursting capacity again. He's a very nice doctor, this Dr. Hogarth. I see a lot of nice doctors. I see a lot of doctors, full stop. I mostly see specialists: neurologists, urologists, ophthalmologists, and so on. My God, I see more doctors than most geriatrics.

I am only thirty-five years old, and if you asked me a few years ago what my life would be like now, a grand tour of London hospitals would not have been included in my answer. If three years ago you told me that I would abruptly leave my home in Long Island, New York, to follow my dreams to London, England, I would have said, 'Wow! Good for me!' If you added, 'You will also be routinely injecting a syringe into your own ass in an effort to slow down an incurable disease you acquired,' I would have said, 'What the fu….'

My name is Marlo Donato Parmelee. I have multiple sclerosis (MS for short). My story is as unique as my name, and yet is it one of two and a half million stories in the world. My story is about a journey within a journey. You see, three years ago, I embarked upon a journey to a new country, a new culture, and a new life. What I didn't realise was that within that, I was embarking upon my greatest and most triumphant journey of all: the journey inside myself.

Little Me

ॐ

I was born and raised in a middle-class suburb on Long Island, New York. My parents, three sisters, and I lived about eighteen miles from Manhattan, benefiting from both the exciting offerings of the metropolis and the soft, sandy beaches of Long Island. It is arguably one of the most desirable places to live in the United States. Even so, I never wanted to stay there permanently. It was too slow for me, for starters. I was always a chick on the move. I had a job since I was fourteen years old. Actually, I had a job when I was thirteen, but my employer fired me when he found out that I had lied about my age. So, against my will, I had to wait until age fourteen to apply for another job. Typical *Marlo stuff.*

Having a payslip with my own name on it has been very important to me as long as I can remember. My parents worked hard to support our family, but financially we always seemed to be just a tad behind most families in our neighbourhood. I think that was because most families at that time had only two or three kids, so money didn't have to stretch as far for them. I worked while I went to university and earned a degree in classical music. I am a singer and a songwriter. I learned early on that making money in music does not happen overnight.

It was during my university years that I got fully swept into the world of the 'day job'. In the same way that actors become waiters, this singer-songwriter somehow became a luxury goods salesperson. It was flexible work and gave me the means to record songs, buy instruments, and continue singing lessons. It also gave me the means to buy designer clothes.

I developed the taste for expensive clothes and accessories early on. Was it hereditary? Maybe. I can't say for sure. My Sicilian grandmother loved expensive clothes. What I can say for sure is that I began collecting pretty things at age seven. I say seven with certainty because I have a picture of me at that age walking in a local parade wearing two-inch pretty heels! I was a Brownie (the younger version of a Girl Scout) with fabulous fashion sense. Every other girl in the picture is wearing trainers or loafers, and there I am hitting the pavement in strappy brown heels! Where my mom bought them, I don't know.

I am what I call 'a girl with pretty things'. I first heard this term while working at Chanel in New York City. One day, a colleague approached me with what I thought was a naughty little question. He had just served a young woman who was dressed head to toe in designer.

'Do you think she has money or just has pretty things?' he asked me. 'I think she only has pretty things,' he continued with a cruel smile.

He felt satisfied believing that she perhaps had less money than him and had just acquired these things the same way we did: staff sales.

That was when I realised that *I* was one of those girls with pretty things. I appreciate designer clothes and shoes. Shoes are a particular weakness for me. I believe a girl can never have too many, and I see nothing wrong with owning duplicates. In fact, owning a backup pair is the sign of ultimate fashion wisdom. How many of us have ruined or worn out a pair of favourite shoes and then wished, even years later that we still had them? That's why you need the backup pair.

Starting in my late teens, I developed other indulgent tastes as well. I went to high school with the kind of girls who went for weekly manicures and pedicures. For me, the ritual started later, in university. At the age of nineteen, I began visiting spas, where I enjoyed all different types of massage and pampering treatments. Discovering the full-body wrap had me hooked for life.

I enjoyed travelling from a young age too, beginning with my first trip to Ireland, when I was seven. I remember feeling as if I *belonged* in Dublin, where my mom had grown up. Visiting all the places she had been when she was a child and young adult opened doors inside my mind. This was probably when the wanderlust inside me was born.

I have always liked trips that were for discovery and trips that were for fun, like my 'tour of every beach we can find on the East Coast' trip when I was twenty. That was a two-week road trip of ten states that I took with my best friend Laura, after watching the film *Thelma and Louise*. We pulled it off with very little planning and a lot of loud music.

Planning holidays was something that I never particularly enjoyed. The older I got, the less I planned and the more money I spent. The hotels I chose got more luxurious and the bathing suits I packed, higher priced. The Bahamas and Las Vegas were two of my favourite getaway spots.

Whilst feeding one of my pricey shopping habits, I met the most perfect specimen of man; my husband. His name is William. He served me in a shop specialising in American Indian merchandise. He too was a salesperson by day and musician by night. Our meeting was fate at its very finest. By the way, ladies and gentlemen, I asked him out on the first date.

The day I met him I had just returned from a holiday I had taken to the Bahamas. I had taken the journey alone. I relaxed, ate in all the best restaurants, went bike riding, and went swimming, all alone. I was happy and secure with myself as a person. I was in a mental state of internal peace and Zen. I felt no need for a boyfriend. So of course, that was the moment I met him.

When I walked into his shop, I was hypnotised by his beautiful eyes. They were brown, almond-shaped, intense eyes. He was tall and slender with thick, long, brown hair. He looked like either a rock star or a vampire. He said 'hello' in a low, shy tone. I felt like falling over.

There's my husband was the first thought that came to mind. It was like I recognised him from a past life; like seeing him *again,* instead of the first time! I bought a dreamcatcher and left the store, immediately phoning Laura.

'Remember I told you yesterday that I was so happy being by myself and that I don't need a guy to make me happy?' I asked her.

'Yeah,' she answered cautiously.

'Now, everything is blown! I just met the guy I am going to marry. I am on my way to your house and *you* are going to help me figure out how to talk to him.'

'Hey, what are you doing out of bed?' she asked. 'Didn't you just have surgery yesterday?'

She was referring to the fact that the day before I had had a noncancerous cyst removed from inside my neck and I had been told to rest for a few days.

'Yes,' I answered. 'So I am not resting! I needed a gift for someone and I am out shopping. Are you my mother?'

'Suit yourself,' she said, well accustomed to my bitchy ways since seventh grade. 'You're a moron. Are you at least wearing a bandage over your stitches?'

'Of course,' I answered. 'And I'm wearing this fabulous leopard-print silk scarf I got last week. You can borrow it if you help me with this. I'm on my way over.'

The following week I was back in his shop, this time with Laura by my side. I browsed the candle section, whilst flashing William my flirtiest eyes. At one point, we stared at each other without speaking and the air in the shop seemed to get thick. I purchased the candles and almost fainted when he counted the change back to me. When Laura and I got outside, I tore off a piece of the bag that my candles were in and wrote him a note on it, asking him out for a drink. I made poor Laura go in with it, as I hid outside like a twenty-four-year-old going on twelve.

He rang me the following day. 'I remember you,' he said. 'You're the girl who bought the candles. You have green eyes.'

'That's me,' I said, trying to keep my composure.

'Yeah, I'll meet you for a drink,' he said. 'Your note impressed me. You're one of the first people I've ever met who isn't too wrapped up in their own bullshit to connect with someone. I'm not going out with you because you're pretty, by the way. If I thought you were ugly I'd go out with you too. I just think you have big balls and I like that in a girl.'

We went out days later and, as they say, the rest was history. The things we had in common went beyond the norm. In one of our first conversations we realised that we each had given our pets the same name! I am not talking about a common name such as 'Fluffy', but 'Sabrina'! William's 'Sabrina' was a Siamese cat and mine was a dog (the prettiest Samoyed).

We found out all kinds of things we had in common from the silly to the serious. We were born in the same hospital, even though we did not live in the same area. The same doctor attended the nursery. We were both vegetarians. We both wrote poetry and music. We both had friends who died in their teens, which made us sensitive to the fragility of life and the constant presence of death. The list went on.

We were the kind of people who believed in fate and looked out for 'signs'. We flew on autopilot most of the time. Instinct was usually our guide. We agreed that life was a grand journey of learning and wondering. We were perfect for each other. We were engaged after three months and married a year after our first meeting in his shop. William, myself, and the two Sabrinas lived as a happy family.

Something Is Missing

ജ

William and I were not like most married couples on Long Island. One difference was that we both had rock bands. My band was called the Marlo Donato Band, and William's band was called Mantis and The Prayer. The bands started off as completely separate projects, but I ended up joining Mantis and the Prayer as a second project. William went through several personnel changes, and by default, I became his keyboard player and back-up singer.

Both bands played many a night at various venues in both New York City and Long Island. We recorded three CDs between us, which we sold at gigs and on the Internet.

By day, I was the assistant store manager of Donna Karan on Long Island. I had moved from Chanel, where I had been for several years, in order to work closer to home and hence have more time for my music. I was dedicated to my role at Donna Karan, but that did not stop me from performing three rehearsals a week and two gigs a month. All my free time was utilised making press kits and building the websites for our bands. I even went back to my Alma Mater for night classes to learn how to use web-creating programs. I went to sleep every night at about1 or 2 a.m. and got up for work at 8 a.m. the next day. My mom used to call me 'the night owl'.

I lived on tea, coffee, and sugar. I had been a vegetarian since I was twenty-two, but other than avoiding meat, I never watched what I ate closely. I ate tons of junk food. I considered chocolate to be a major food group, especially 'good' chocolate. Well, OK, I *still* think it's good for you.

Another thing that made William and me different from other married couples was that we did not want the typical 'American Dream'. The thought of having children and living in a big house with a white picket fence made us cringe.

While most young couples on Long Island were saving for a down payment on their first home, we put all of our money into CDs, websites, promotional materials, mailing, and so on. Owning a house did not matter to us. Having children did not matter to us. Only music mattered to us. One by one, our friends were getting married and having babies. Girlfriends would say, 'I'm pregnant again,' and I'd say, 'We recorded another CD!' Songs were our babies.

Despite not wanting children, we were in no way ostracised by these friends. Most of them, if not all of them, loved the idea that we were still pursuing our dreams, despite the odds being against us. We often had our friends and family at our apartment for dinners and live entertainment.

We didn't live like starving artists. We lived in a very pleasant, safe neighbourhood. Leaving our car unlocked or the windows down was not a concern. Our apartment was lovely. We had all the amenities to make life easier: a double-load washing machine, dryer, dishwasher, and air conditioning.

We were a train ride away from Manhattan, so we were there all the time, not just for gigs or shopping. It was not uncommon for William to get a midnight craving for his favourite food, falafel, which had to be from one particular place on MacDougal Street in Greenwich Village. He would always coax me into driving in with him to get it. My best memories of this include driving over the Manhattan Bridge, looking at the illuminated Twin Towers, and singing songs we made up about falafel balls and hot sauce.

We had a good life, a fun life. Our life was about having lots of laughs, music, and freedom. We were on a journey of learning and creating art. We felt that the journey would take us anywhere we wanted to go.

In 2002, William and I were getting bored of New York and were talking more and more about moving somewhere else. Our Long Island life was getting too comfortable, and we were not challenged enough spiritually or artistically. Something was missing. We both had a growing wanderlust and big dreams. We had to do something drastic about it.

That year, we planned a holiday to London to sightsee and visit my cousin, whom I had not seen since I was a teenager. William and I thought it would be 'cool' to bring a guitar with us and try to play some open-mic nights. Certain nights of the week, some clubs give an opportunity for anyone to come up and play a couple of songs. You go early in the night and sign up to play on a first-come, first-served basis. I researched on the Internet some clubs that had an open-mic night in London, so we would not be entirely lost when we arrived.

On the plane over, I told William about my previous trip to London when I was sixteen. Back then I had fallen in love with the city. The thought of walking around Piccadilly Circus again made my pulse quicken with excitement. My intuition told me that this would be no ordinary holiday. I told him that if he really liked London, than maybe we should just pack up and move. He was laughing, but William was as spontaneous as I was, and I could see in his eyes that he would consider the idea.

We talked about our disenchantment with the music scene in New York. We agreed that people there were not receptive to many different types of music. William's music at the time had a strong retro vibe, and we felt that not enough people appreciated it.

I wrote more pop-oriented music, but I felt like that wasn't always appreciated either, especially by the managers and promoters at the venues we played. I remember walking around NYC, handing out press kits to club after club. Most of the managers had such bad attitudes. One manager of a very well known club in Greenwich Village actually sat on a chair outside the venue while he played the guitar, asking us about our music. He never looked up from his guitar the whole time we spoke. It was creepy. He also didn't seem to like the fact that we were from Long Island, as he noticeably stopped listening to us the second we mentioned it.

Another manager looked patronizingly at me and said, 'What kind of music do you play, *honey?*'

'I play pop-rock,' I answered. 'All original....'

He cut me off quickly. 'We don't do pop here, *sweetheart*. We book heavier acts.'

I was tired of hearing that kind of response. The clubs on Long Island also played a lot of heavy music. On the other end of the spectrum, many played just acoustic music. I felt as if I didn't quite fit into any scene. William didn't either.

It wasn't all black and white, though. Despite our feeling of not fitting in, we had some minor successes. Both of us were played and interviewed on local radio, and both of us became members of ASCAP (American Society of Composers and Publishers). Sometimes we'd feel confused because we would have a terrific gig where strangers (as opposed to family and friends) would buy our CDs and rave about the performance. But in spite of all this, we knew we needed to be where people were more open-minded and less uptight. We didn't know where that was, but it certainly wasn't New York.

After a few nights in London, William had fallen in love with the city too. We played two small venues and found that we preferred playing in London. OK, it was only two venues, but the energy was fantastic, and people seemed to appreciate a greater variety of music than they did in New York.

The club managers were much nicer than the ones in New York. We phoned several of them, and they would say things like, 'What kind of music do you play, mate?' When we answered, they always said something like, 'Let's hear it!' The response was more open. If we were going to make a living in the music business, it would happen in London. If we moved to London, we would be out of our comfortable Long Island life and therefore force ourselves to create the life we wanted.

On the plane back to New York, I asked William, 'So, what do you think?'

'Let's do it,' he said. 'Let's pack our things!'

'Are you serious?' I asked, my enthusiasm growing.

He smiled at me. 'Are you?'

'We'll have to figure out how we can legally live in England,' I said.

'Yes,' he said. 'Let's research that as soon as we get home. We'll make it happen. We have to follow our dreams, Marlo. We need to be shaken up, pulled out of our cosy life. Life is too short.'

'Yes,' I agreed. 'We both know that's true.'

'We have nothing to lose,' he said.

'No, just our minds,' I laughed. 'Oh, and maybe money. Yes, nothing to lose....'

Weeks later, we were standing in the Irish Consulate in NYC, hearing the woman behind the counter tell us that I was born an Irish citizen.

'Sorry, what?' I asked, making her repeat it.

Because my mom was born in Ireland and moved to the United States during a specific time period, I was born both an Irish *and* American citizen: a *dual citizen*! As odd as it sounds, I never knew I was a dual citizen until that moment. My mom did not know either. She had become an American citizen many years before. Her children were born in the United States and therefore were only American as far as she was concerned.

Having dual citizenship meant that I could live and work in any country that was part of the European Union (EU). The joy I felt made me want to lean over and hug the woman behind the counter. The excitement at the Irish Consulate was only surpassed months later, when we left the British Consulate, where we were informed that since William was married to an Irish citizen, then he was entitled to a visa to live and work in the EU as well!

The sun was beating down on us when we marched out of that consulate building. We literally skipped and hopped down Third Avenue screaming and singing! We sang in the street, making up camp songs about 'our adventure'. We finally calmed down when we got on the train back to Long Island. We fell into a seat and smiled at each other.

'Holy shit,' I said. 'We are so outta here.'

The Big Move

~

We left New York in a huge snowstorm, on St. Patrick's Day, 2004. We thought that would be the luckiest possible day to begin the adventure. We arrived at Heathrow Airport on the 18th of March. Our first two months of living in London did not go as smoothly as we had envisioned. In fact, those first two months were hell.

The British pound was killing the American dollar at an exchange rate of $1.86 to the pound, so we felt like we lost half our money straight away. We knew the exchange rates were not in our favour when we moved. We had prepared for this, but mentally, it was upsetting to see half of our total life savings seemingly disappear. Our $10,000 that we exchanged was now a £5,400 cheque that we carried around (literally in a pocket) for two weeks.

Why did we carry it? Contrary to what I was told before the move, no bank in London would let us open an account because we did not have a UK address or a utility bill. (Incidentally, you can't rent a flat without a bank account. You do the math!) We brought with us every bank statement we ever had, but we could not open a damn account.

William carried the cheque in his pocket because we were afraid to leave it in the flat we were staying at. Until we found our own flat, we were lodging with my wonderful auntie in a council flat on the outskirts of London. We had visited her before and had not comprehended the realities of the neighbourhood she lived in. Visiting is never the same as living somewhere.

The neighbourhood was a rough, gang-ridden area. My auntie had been burgled twice, once whilst she was actually at home. There was police activity during all hours of the day and night. We were awakened on several nights by screams and shouts, followed by police sirens.

There was a boy murdered across the street two days after our arrival. At the bus stop where we would begin the hour-long ride into London city each day, there was a disturbing sign posted up, reading 'MURDER'. The sign was about three feet tall and the letters were gigantic.

'Oh my God! What the hell is this?' I asked William when we first saw it.

'We're not in Kansas anymore,' he answered and grabbed my hand.

We took a closer look at the sign. It had a picture of the handsome murdered boy, who was seventeen years old. He had been shot *and* stabbed. The police were asking if anyone had information.

'Where the hell are we living?' I mumbled. It affected me deeply.

Longing to go back to our safe little Long Island neighbourhood, I cried in William's arms every single night for two weeks. I wanted to go home. I felt that maybe we had made a mistake. The only thing that kept us in London was the innate reaction to stay and fight for our dream. We had wanted so badly to move here and create a new life. Not to mention that I had told every friend I ever had that I was moving here to start this great new life. I do have a great deal of pride, you know. We could not just fold up. Nothing was going to stop us. Besides, London did have a Starbucks on every fifth corner, so how bad could it be?

Walking through a half dozen London neighbourhoods, we searched for a flat. The Internet research that I conducted for several months before the trip only got us so far. The rest was legwork. I have never walked so much in my life. We learned many of the streets of London in our first two weeks. I did not realise how much walking we were going to do, and of course, I had packed all the wrong shoes. We walked every day for hours upon hours, from morning until night. We set out on the first day of flat hunting, looking like two chic New Yorkers having a stroll. By the fifth or sixth day, we were looking like two gypsies desperate for food and shelter. Every night we returned to my auntie's house sore and broken, ravenous for the gigantic dinners she would lovingly make us before sending us off to bed.

We visited so many estate agents, it was hard to keep track. We saw flat after flat, until finally, on the tenth day, we found our cute home in Clapham. It was a small, furnished one-bedroom flat. It had minimal amenities, but it did have a little balcony that had a view of Clapham Common. We moved in on the 1st of April. Yes, *April Fool's Day!*

I started working a few days later. This was one aspect of the move that I planned fairly well. While still in New York, I had arranged an interview with a recruiter here in London. He put me in touch with a designer label on Old Bond Street that shall remain nameless, since I ended up hating it. I interviewed there on the 20th of March and again on the 23rd. The label hired me days after and I became its ladies department manager.

Once again, things did not go as I expected. The company was a disaster. I had a staff of ten people, most of them from Italy. They were adorable, and I fell in love with them instantly. At times, I felt like their foster mother. They were good people. Unfortunately, we were all attracted to a company with great designs but no management to back it up.

Nothing was in order in the store. There was no proper documentation of inventory. There was no proper documentation of clients. There was just no management from store level on up to the CEO, and no one seemed to care. They just wanted me to look sexy and sell dresses, nothing more.

I had a tight button-down blouse that I wore as my uniform. My manager told me to unbutton a few buttons and show off my breasts a little. This might seem appalling to people who have not worked in the fashion industry. It might even seem like a lawsuit ready to happen. For me, though, it was just more of a fashion concern. As I was also given rosary beads to wear around my neck, I felt the look was a little too '1980s Madonna'.

I wore it, though, and tried to just be content that we were selling so many dresses. I couldn't be content, though. The degree of disorganisation was mounting and no one allowed me to change it. Very often, a team of merchandisers would come to the store to set up displays. Unlike at most luxury retail shops, the merchandising could not be done during hours that were open to the public. Why? That was just the company rule. So, instead, I had to stay at night while they changed the store around endlessly.

The team came without plans each time. They would move everything around and then discuss in Italian what they didn't like. Then they would move it all back! I do speak a little Italian, but I could only understand parts of what they were saying. It was very upsetting.

Because of these disorganised merchandising nights, I was starting to work fifteen-hour days, without any extra compensation. The store manager told me that she was glad she hired me, because now she did not have to be the one to stay with them. Isn't that sweet?

Despite the unacceptable levels of dysfunction within the company, sales were soaring. The clothes sold themselves. If you wanted to be sexy, this was the label you wanted to wear. Any famous singer, model, or actress worth their salt has worn this label, and many of these people were clients of this particular shop. In fact, this shop had two regular visitors from the pop and football worlds. They were at one time considered the 'King and Queen of England'. Even the prospects of *them* visiting did not excite me.

It was all overshadowed by stress and exhaustion, which were quickly becoming major parts of my daily life. The nonsense at work was cutting into my personal time and making me too tired to play my keyboard when I got home. Instead of supplementing my music career, my job was draining me. I had no time to think about my music. I was miserable.

The Signs Begin

ເວ

It was during these extremely stressful first weeks of work that I noticed the big toe on my left foot was numb. The reason for this was clear to me: I blamed the company's pointy shoes. They had given me two pairs of free shoes for my uniform. They were obviously trying to destroy my precious, pampered feet! The shoes that season were excessively pointy and, evidently, were cutting off my circulation. Even my three-inch-heel 'walking' boots were pointy. I thought that the right thing to do was to stop wearing all the pointy shoes, but the thought of a round toe that season was too much to stomach. My fashionista self mused, *The season is almost over. I will only have to suffer for a couple more months. Looking good sometimes requires pain.*

At night I would soak my feet in the tub and try to rub feeling back into the toe. I am a person who always took care of my feet: they were pampered and pedicured at all times. I never had dry heels or an ugly toe. Never!

As the price of a pedicure in London was ridiculously expensive, I started giving myself pedicures at home. It was during one of these pedicures that I realised just how extreme my toe numbness was. I polished my big toenail but could not feel the brush glide across it. It was like painting someone else's nail. It looked like mine, but somehow it wasn't. The feeling disturbed me. I envisioned painting a dead person's toe. Disgusting!

The feeling was much more intense than the usual toe numbness that comes from wearing uncomfortable shoes. I took out my pumice stone and started rubbing the toe furiously with it. I could barely feel it! *What the hell is going on?* I thought. *What, did you just up and die?* I asked the toe telepathically. *But why are you not blue or black?* I was confused. I called William in to look at it.

'Watch this,' I said and began banging it harshly with the pumice stone. 'I can't feel a thing, even if I bang it hard! I cannot feel anything!'

'Stop doing that,' he said angrily. 'Why don't you stop wearing those damn shoes?'

'Guys don't get it,' I explained. 'Do you know how many times I have had to soak my feet for days because I wore high heels to impress someone at a dance? We girls learn masochism from an early age. Heels look great, William. You know it. You can't expect to walk on a tilt and not experience at least some form of pain or numbness.' OK, this was more numbness than what should be normal. I admit that now.

Despite my efforts to ignore the problem, I was becoming concerned. The situation was bad enough for me to experiment with boring, flatter shoes (though they were Chanel). For the next week, I did not wear the pointy shoes. I wore round-toe flat shoes at work and trainers when I was not working.

I had rarely worn trainers in my life. I hated how they looked, but I went to Oxford Street and bought my first pair of proper British trainers. British trainers look better than big white American sneakers, in my opinion. They are sleeker, daintier. My new shoes were thin and black with white stripes. I was certain they would be my remedy, but after days of wearing them, it became clear that they were not the remedy I had hoped them to be. The numbness in fact, seemed to have increased. I thought this must be from the damage I had already caused, and I assessed that it would probably take months for the feeling to come back.

As more days went by, my toe remained dead. There was literally no feeling. My blasé reaction was turning to fear, but I continued doing nothing about my toe. I learned to ignore it; partly because I was working such long hours that I did not mentally have time to deal with it.

I never thought about going to the doctor. My problem seemed petty. 'Hi, Doctor, my toe is numb, got any pills?' Besides, I had convinced myself of the reason for the toe's death: masochistic shoe wearing. I had no idea that the numb toe was one of the first signs that lesions were forming on my brain. I was utterly oblivious to the massacre that was happening inside my own brain.

&

About a month after I noticed my numb toe, the next telltale sign of MS reared its ugly head. One May morning while I was brushing my teeth, I noticed that the bathroom mirror looked odd. It looked like it was warped. I could not put my finger on the exact problem, but the mirror did not look right.

'William, look at this!' I called. 'Our bathroom mirror is warped. What a cheap piece of crap! Look, do you see it?'

'I don't see anything,' he said, coming into the bathroom behind me. 'It looks like it always does.'

I remember worrying that there must be something wrong with him. How could he not see that our mirror was warped when it was so blatant? I was puzzled. I started to get a little angry with him. Was he joking? Was he crazy?

'The mirror is definitely warped,' I said irritably. 'Look at it again. You'll see it.'

He left the bathroom, shaking his head, while I continued studying the mirror from several different angles. As I looked at it longer, it seemed to become normal again. Was I losing my mind? Perhaps *I* was the one who was crazy. Maybe I was just tired. I did feel particularly drained that morning. I finally shrugged it off and continued my routine as usual.

Later that morning, we went to Canary Wharf, where William had a meeting with Citibank. We had been in London for over five weeks, and all of William's job offers were falling through. Companies did not think he was a reliable candidate because they thought he would leave after his visa expired in a year.

Some even got confused and did not understand that William had the right to work in the UK because he was married to an Irish citizen. One company actually apologised to William after hiring someone else for the position he was interviewing for, saying, 'Sorry, we now realise that you *can* indeed work in the UK, but we already filled the position while we were waiting to hear from our legal department.'

William had spent the past couple of weeks waiting tables at a local Mexican restaurant and he hated it. We were frustrated, but we thought this next meeting would change all of that. The initial contact person at Citibank seemed to understand that William could work in the UK.

I knew he would be in the meeting for a long time, so I told him I would shop at the mall there, and we would meet up in two hours at the newspaper stand near the tube entrance. Meeting at the exact time was very important because we only had one mobile phone between us, and William had it, in case he had to ring the interviewer.

We went our separate ways. I went to see what shops were in the mall. There was a large Boots the Chemist. I can always do major shopping at a store like that. I bought body cream, facial scrub, nail polish: tons of things I did not need. I even applied for the Boots shopper card. Now I was becoming a proper Londoner. I was excited.

I browsed through shop after shop, enjoying every minute, except that I began to feel very tired. As I walked into maybe the tenth store, I started to feel a little light-headed as well. As I continued walking, the feeling increased. It did not feel as if I was going to pass out. I had felt that before. This was more like a feeling of coming out of my body, as if it was not mine. I felt detached from myself and everything else. I knew I should sit, but I could not find a seat inside the mall, no matter how hard I looked.

When I looked in certain directions, things did not look normal. They looked slightly out of focus. Certain objects that I looked at seemed to tilt upwards. Something was severely wrong with my vision, although it was hard to pinpoint until I got outside the mall.

I made my way outside, thinking the fresh air would help me. It had started to rain, making everything look more blurry. Suddenly, the raindrops looked as if they were swinging and tilting. I could not believe what I was seeing. I kept wiping my eyes.

As I tried to focus, a feeling in my head like bubbles popping came over me. The bubbles were floating around inside my skull. I imagined myself as a shaken champagne bottle whose cork was about to pop. It was not painful, but it was intense.

I couldn't understand what was happening. *I was shopping happily ten minutes ago; why have I stepped into a Salvador Dali painting?* Passers-by looked cloudy and seemed to smear into one another. My thoughts raced with fear. *Oh my God, I am having a heart attack. No, I don't have pain in my chest. This is a stroke. I am having a stroke!*

My head also felt as if it weighed as much as the rest of my body. I kept praying that I would not collapse in the middle of Canary Wharf. I did not have any identification on me apart from credit cards. I stumbled to our designated meeting spot. I thought, *If I collapse here on the ground, who will tell William? No one. He will probably return to this spot, and I'd have been carted off in an ambulance already.* I became panic stricken. I was so overwhelmed by these feelings that I could no longer stay. I rushed inside a building and slumped down on a bench that was located right in front of the glass doors. I thought that if I was going to collapse, I would be safer indoors.

From the bench, I had a partial view of our meeting spot, so I was certain that I would see William or a smeared version of him when he arrived there. I closed my eyes for a few minutes and tried to concentrate on feeling better. I drank some water. I told myself to pull it together.

Getting sick is not an option right now. William needs my support today. I kept looking in the direction where I expected to see him after the interview.

I never saw him.

William waited and waited. It took me probably forty minutes to begin recovering from the strange episode. The weird feeling started to lessen and my vision came back into focus. It did not return to normal, but it was good enough to enable me to get up off the bench.

By the time I pulled myself together and went outside, William had been waiting for a long time and was not happy.

'Where the hell were you?'

'I was busy going blind,' I replied. 'I think I might have had a stroke.'

He looked at my shopping bags in disbelief. (It was also not the first time I had been late due to heavy shopping activity.)

'I am not kidding,' I said. 'Something is wrong with me.'

He looked confused. Here I was telling him that some medical trauma had just happened to me and yet I looked completely fine. I was confused too. It was difficult to describe the feeling I had in my head.

'Forget it,' I said. 'I felt sick, but I feel better now.'

As we started on our way back home, the weird feeling in my head continued to lessen. Something was still off, but I couldn't quite verbalise what it was. My vision was ever-so-slightly blurry. William assumed that I was fine and began telling me about the interview. I found it difficult to concentrate on what he was saying. I could see his mouth moving, but couldn't really differentiate between his words and the background noise of the other people around us. I seemed to be encapsulated in my own little world. I felt so drained after my whole ordeal. All I could think about was sleeping.

On the train home, I tried to think of more reasons why this could have happened to me. I figured that I must have been dehydrated or hungry. Maybe I had eaten something bad recently. I couldn't remember what I had eaten that morning. Whatever it was that happened scared the hell out of me. I knew somewhere in the back of my mind that this was not a good sign, but I convinced myself that I was dehydrated and overtired. I told myself that I would feel better later.

When we arrived back at our flat, I got straight into bed. I was completely exhausted and traumatised. I hoped that I would never feel that way again. Sadly, that feeling, and worse, would soon return for a long stay.

The next day, I went into work feeling like I hadn't slept for weeks. I was exceptionally tired, but that was nothing new for me. *When you are working fifteen-hour days, you should be tired,* I reasoned with myself.

I noticed that morning that things looked slightly blurry when I looked to the right. It was hard to determine what exactly the problem was, but it was definitely different from whatever it was that had happened to me the previous day.

In retrospect, I was in denial because I did not put the two problems together. What had happened the day before was something totally separate. I continued my day and tried not to look to the right. It was very annoying. What was going on? I started to think, *Obviously, I must need glasses.* I had always had 20/20 vision, but I assumed that my vision might have changed overnight. *At least I made it thirty-one years with perfect vision*, I thought, trying to see the bright side.

After work that day, I ran from my job on Old Bond Street to Oxford Street, where there are many eyeglass stores. These are the kind of stores where a technician gives you a quick eye exam and you get your glasses the same day.

I got my exam, and it was easy for me. I was able to see everything on the chart, including the tiniest writing, which surprised me. I still seemed to have 20/20 vision.

I explained to the technician the worrying things that were happening to me. She did not seem to have an answer, so I tried to come up with my own answers for her. I told her that my computer screen at work was in an awkward position, so that I had to look down at it. Could the act of constantly looking down at a computer screen give me these weird symptoms?

She told me that constantly looking downward at a screen is not healthy, and that if I could not change the position of the screen, then I should rest my eyes every so often. She also said that stress could affect one's vision. I agreed with her and told her that I was extremely stressed lately.

'Try to relax,' she suggested. 'You might want to come back in a few months if things do not improve.'

She gave me a prescription for antiglare eyeglasses that I should wear at the computer.

Between the glasses and the relaxing that I swore to myself that I would soon partake in (as if), I was sure I would start to feel better. *Yes,* I thought. *A chic pair of Fendi glasses, and I will be cured!* I was so happy! I could not wait to tell William that it was because of stress, coupled with the computer at work, that my vision was poor. It made sense to me.

Over the next few days, I wore my beautiful glasses while I was at the computer. I actually had myself convinced that they were working. The truth was they were not working, and after a week of wearing them, I had to admit that my vision was still not normal. I was again down on my luck and out £200.

In the days after my eyeglass defeat, I was on an emotional downslide. My vision slowly and steadily worsened. Things looked out of focus but then started to slightly double as well. This worsened further when I looked to the extreme right, especially if I was looking in the distance as well.

I usually took a bus and the tube to work. On one particular day, I was walking to the bus stop and I began to feel like I was floating as I walked. It did not feel good. I felt like the bubbles were exploding in my head again. I looked at other people waiting at the bus stop. Could they see that something was wrong? Did I look off? Apparently I looked normal, because a girl stopped to ask me directions. This always happens to me. No matter what city I am in, whether I know my way around or not, people always ask me for directions. I was born with an invisible sign that says, 'Need directions? Ask me!'

'Excuse me,' she said. 'Is the college on this road?'

'Yes,' I answered, drawing from memory where it was. I pointed. 'Do you see that building over there?'

'Yes,' she answered.

Good, I thought. *Because I actually can't really see it today. What the hell?*

'Just turn right at that building and you'll see it on your left.'

I rubbed my eyes. I couldn't figure out what my visual problem was until the bus approached. As I watched it get nearer, it looked out of focus, almost like a haze was over it. It was also slightly doubled. To describe it accurately, I would have to say that it looked like it was just coming out of itself. It was almost one image, but not quite. It was weird. Imagine looking at two negatives of the same picture. Now imagine superimposing one on top of the other. Pretend, if you will, that you took one of those negatives and shifted it a centimetre to the right. This is what the bus looked like.

As the bus got closer, it also looked like its wheels were coming off the road, like it might take off in flight! It was like living in a version of *Chitty, Chitty, Bang, Bang!*

It sounds scary, but that day I was almost more fascinated than scared. I also think I was too unaware to be frightened. In fact, I thought I was pretty much invincible back then.

Trapped in total denial, I functioned like that for days longer, and things got increasingly worse. Crossing the street became a danger. I could not see cars coming if I looked to the right, and in England, you must always look to the right. The situation was fast becoming a nightmare.

Against William's pleas, I refused to see a doctor. I had myself convinced that stress was the cause, so there was no need to see a doctor. Everyone whom I talked to at work seemed to agree with me. That is a clever way to diagnose something. Tell four or five people your problem and get them to agree with your own diagnosis. It makes you feel a lot better.

I didn't look ill, or so I thought. William thought my eyes looked glassy and dark. I thought I looked like a tired version of my usually fabulous self. I had to wear much more concealer under my eyes than I usually did, but so what?

Looking back at pictures of myself taken during that time, I now realise that I did not look well at all. My eyes were extremely blackened and glazed. They were what my mom would call 'in the back of my head'. I basically looked like shit.

One night during all of this, I remembered something. A couple of weeks prior, something flew in my eye as my train pulled into the station. I immediately told William, who did not quite 'buy' any of my stories that I made up regarding how my eye problems began.

'No, Marlo. Something is really wrong,' he argued.

'No! *This* is it!' I insisted. 'Something flew in my eye and it must have stuck there! It is probably a tiny piece of metal! I just have to flush it out with water!'

I started rinsing my eye with water. I was in the bathroom for a long time that night because things got even worse. It is amazing how fast one problem can turn into two.

The eye flushing became toilet flushing. While I was busy with my eye, a bladder infection was starting. I had been prone to these infections for the past several years. I would get them quite severely. One moment, I felt a tingle when I peed, and a half-hour later, I'd be urinating thick blood. For this reason, I carried antibiotics with me at all times.

I felt the usual signs of the infection coming. This included pain in my abdomen, chills, and the urge to pee immediately. I knew it was coming on strongly, so I got my stash of antibiotics and said a little prayer for myself.

The sting of the actual urination was horrific. As anyone who has ever had it knows, you feel like you need to pee a gallon of liquid. What comes out? One tiny, excruciating drop. Then a chill rides up through your body, taking your mind off the pain that is in your abdomen. Seconds later, you feel the same sensation and go through the whole thing again. To me, it is one of the worst maladies a person can have. That night became a real drama.

A & E and a Curry

❧

The next day, I woke up feeling worse than ever. I stupidly dragged myself into work. Everyone asked how my eye was. I told them it was the same. I did not even mention the bladder infection because I didn't want them to think that the new manager was totally falling apart. Besides, I still wanted to believe that nothing was wrong, even though I knew I was not well. I was deep in denial land.

That day, I was telling the store manager that I thought something had flown in my eye. She told me that there was a very good eye hospital in London, called Moorfields. She told me that the skilled doctors there had helped her son a few years before. They only take care of eyes, and they have a fantastic reputation. She informed me that Moorfields had an emergency department that was open all night.

If something were in my eye that would be the place to get it out.

Finally, I thought. *I have to end this! I will go tonight and get this piece of metal out of my eye. They will fix me.*

After work, William took me to Moorfields Eye Hospital on City Road. We took the tube to Old Street Station. When the train pulled into that station, the on-board announcement rang out loudly, 'Alight here for Moorfields Eye Hospital.' I thought that was great.

'That's where they are going to fix my eye,' I said to William, playfully.

'Yes,' he said. 'Let's *alight* here!'

The first thing that impressed me about Moorfields was something that was not even in the hospital: It was in the tube stop. When you arrive at Old Street tube station, there is a sign that tells you which way to exit to get to the hospital. When you get to that exit, there is a green line on the ground that leads you to the hospital doors! It was very *Wizard of Oz*!

'Follow the *green* brick road,' William sang. 'This is impressive,' he continued when he stopped singing. 'They obviously take helping visually impaired people very seriously.'

The waiting room at Accident and Emergency (A&E) was packed with problem eyes. I was shocked that this many people could have eye ailments. It looked like a war zone. There were people with eyepatches, bandages: you name it. People had swollen eyes, bulging eyes, red eyes, turned eyes—and those were just the doctors. Just kidding. Seriously, though, it *did* look like a war zone.

A nurse told us that there was a three-hour wait and said that we could go outside and get dinner if we wanted. We left the emergency room and ate at an Indian restaurant down the road. It was a good discovery for us, as we went back there many times in the years to follow.

We laughed through the whole dinner, thinking of our circumstances. When the waiter asked if we wanted dessert, something we rarely turn down, we were forced to say no. We had to remember that we were not really out to a leisurely dinner. We were really in a queue at the hospital up the road.

We thought it was comical. We were enjoying ourselves. I don't think either of us thought that I had a life altering problem. They were going to flush my eye out, and I would be fine. It would just be another crazy night in London.

We arrived back to A & E just in time. They were calling my name. Various technicians performed all kinds of eye tests on me, and I passed all of them. I still had 20/20 vision, so I was reading the smallest letters on the eye chart.

It was especially easy because they had me cover one eye. I would later find out that my vision was distorted only when the two eyes were open. After the initial tests, a nurse put dilating drops in my eyes and told us to wait in the waiting room again.

By this time, the war zone had filled up even more, and there were no seats available except for a row in the children's waiting area. William smiled at me as he guided me to a chair surrounded by toys and colouring books.

While we were sitting there, we heard a voice coming from behind a curtain. It was a doctor asking a patient where he works and how he got this piece of metal in his eye. She was removing it.

'Keep your head completely still,' she told him in a cold, stern tone. 'You must not move!' Her manner was a little too stern for my taste. 'Stay still!' she reprimanded.

I imagined a terrified patient, shaking in his seat. I started feeling very nervous for him. I felt ill listening to the conversation. I slowly realised from the dialogue that if debris is in your eye, they don't flush it out with an eyecup, as I had hoped. Instead, they go in with tiny tweezers! This was a sickening thought!

I continued listening to the whole scenario and imagining the horrors taking place behind that curtain. I started anticipating *my* turn with the doctor. She would try to put the tweezers in my eye and would become increasingly angry when I couldn't keep my head still. She would call over two oversized attendants who would hold me in a headlock while she went for my eye!

I was sure that this was what would happen to me, and I got increasingly anxious.

When I am nervous, I usually start giggling. I am a person who laughs a lot, anyway. Sometimes people ask me why I laugh so much and I tell them that I am smiling out loud. I also happen to find humour in almost everything that life throws at me.

I started one of my usual laughing fits, and tears soon began dripping down my face. I did not want the staff to see me laughing, as they would think I wasn't taking my visit seriously. I tried to remain solemn, but my attempts were futile. I was now shaking with laughter, while William squeezed my hand, signalling me to control myself.

'Don't start doing this,' he warned. 'If you don't stop, I'll start.'

I answered him manically. 'I am going to start playing with the toys now, Daddy.'

'Stop it, please,' he pleaded, but he started to crack a smile.

'Do you dare me to sit on the floor and start screaming the ABCs at the top of my lungs?' I asked.

'Fine,' he said. 'Do it. I dare you.'

I felt crazy at that moment. My nerves were shot. I was riddled with fear. I thought it would have been more appropriate if I were waiting in a mental hospital. That thought provoked me to start laughing even harder, if that was possible. I was a wreck!

'You really need to stop now,' William said. I looked at him and he started laughing hard. He was on the verge of the insanity also. It got more and more out of control. We could not stop for the world.

I said in a loud drunken-like whisper, 'If my friends could see me now!' I started gasping for air, as I continued. 'How is London, Marlo? It's great! I hate my job. I am urinating blood and going blind and it has only been a couple of months! I'm having a fantastic time!'

We were convulsing with laughter. The laughter came to a screeching halt when a doctor called my name. It wasn't the lady doctor who performed the metal removal from behind the curtain, but I still wanted to run.

The doctor examined my eyes closely and said that my right eye had some small inflammation behind it, but there were no particles in it. I thought this was great news, because now I would not have to endure those tweezers. He took my temperature. I had a fever, which surprised me because I didn't feel warm. He told me the temperature in Celsius, which at the time I did not understand. I only knew temperature in Fahrenheit, as Americans learn it. I just nodded, as if I understood.

He asked me if anything else bothered me. I told him that I had a bladder infection and was taking antibiotics.

'Anything else?' he asked.

'Nothing else bothers me,' I told him. The thought of mentioning my numb toe never crossed my mind. William was sitting in the room with us, and it never crossed his mind either.

'It looks like you have a viral infection,' the doctor concluded. 'It can manifest anywhere in the body, in your case, in your bladder and your eyes.' He told me to take Ibuprofen for the swelling behind the eye. He said that I should take it for the next couple of weeks, and the problem should clear up.

I left the hospital thinking that I would never have to go there again. Little did I know that in the near future I would be back so many times, it would become my second home.

My eye problem took approximately five more weeks to completely go away. Three of those weeks were pure misery, in which my eyes began to pain me. At times, the pain was an unbearable dull ache from hell. I felt like my eyes were being held in vice grips. Turning them to look to the side was torture. I simply stopped turning them one day. I started to adjust with robotic head movements.

My head felt different too. The feeling of bubbles exploding was present most of the time and it was becoming overwhelming. I felt like I was walking around in my very own bubble. I did not feel like myself. I just felt out of sorts.

For weeks I could not even cross the street by myself. I was terrified of crossing. For my whole adult life, I had crossed busy streets against the light or had run between cars with a coffee in one hand and my mobile phone in the other. Now, jaywalking was out of the question.

I adapted a little trick to cross the road. I would stand behind elderly people and wait for them to cross. This was a useful trick, as they would not leave the curb unless there was plenty of time to get across to the other side.

Sometimes the elderly people and I would be waiting at the curb for a long time while no cars went by. For this reason, I had to take my little 'trick' one step further. To look like I was waiting for a good reason, I would pretend I was searching for something in my handbag. *Hmm, where did I put that piece of something or other? Oh look! The light just changed. I'll have to look for it later.*

I really had to be careful crossing the street when there were no elderly people around. I would have to look for my next group of people: mothers with small children. They took more chances than my elderly crossing guards, but they were still pretty careful. If they weren't around, I was really screwed.

It was during this time that I started to think carefully about what panties I put on in the morning in case I did get run over later in the day. I didn't want my body to be found in the street with worn knickers. Every morning I would choose my bra and panties while saying out loud, 'Yes, I could be found dead in these.' As amusing as it sounds, it was terrifying. It did not stop me though. I never once stayed home. Every day, I made myself keep going.

Riding the trains was a nightmare. I would sometimes shut one eye while going down the steps to the tube. I had to hold on to the rail for dear life. This slowed me down, but I was already moving at a slower pace than normal anyway. I held up the flow of people traffic. I had now become one of the people whom I used to whiz by.

Whilst on the train, I would hold on to the pole and just close my eyes altogether. Getting a seat during rush hour was usually not an option, but when I did get one, I would shout, *Thank you God!* inside my head.

All of this travelling on public transportation certainly was an ordeal, but I never thought about finding another mode of transport. It was simply not an option. I had a viral infection, and this was part of the misery associated with it.

Focusing my thoughts was also difficult during those five weeks. The feelings in my head were always bothersome. I constantly had loud subtexts conversing in my mind as well. Whilst talking to colleagues or clients I had to use extra energy to concentrate on them. I wanted to say, 'I'm sorry, can we continue this conversation next week, or maybe next month?

Hopefully, by then, I won't feel like *Alice in Wonderland*. I'm a bit fucked up right now.'

I would try to keep people to the left side of me, so that I could see them better. That only helped a little, not to mention that it was exhausting trying to dance around to the right side of people all the time.

It was so hard to function under these conditions. I got tired of conducting myself as if nothing was wrong. I was constantly pretending, like a drunken teenager trying to act sober in front of her parents. It was draining in every way.

Functioning was much easier in front of William. He was the only person that I didn't have to act in front of. I could relax with him. Even so, it was hard to listen to him when he was speaking. My concentration was nonexistent at that point. William's words were becoming background noise. My noisy subtext and head bubbles were taking up the foreground every night. Most evenings I could only stay up until 10 p.m., compared to my usual bedtime of 1 a.m. I had no interest in sex of any kind. As far as I was concerned, my mind and my vagina were closed for business.

This was the problem that really got William's attention. He suggested many times that I take off from work and see a doctor again.

'It's been much more than two weeks,' he kept saying. He was referring to the eye problems and subconsciously the sex.

'That doctor at Moorfields said your eyes should be better by now.'

He was right. I should have gone back to the doctor. In fact, the hospital rang me to schedule a follow-up visit, and I did not make an appointment. I was stubborn. I figured that the 'virus' was just taking a long time to go away. I still thought that stress played a huge role in my symptoms.

'I have to relieve myself of stress if I am going to get better,' I told William one night.

'Good,' he said. 'Why don't you start by quitting your job? We came here to follow our dreams and you are not following yours, are you?'

He was right.

I handed in my notice days later. I could not stay at a job that made me so unhappy and stressed. I could not see myself working unnecessarily long days anymore, especially whilst dressed like Madonna from the Eighties. I did not come to London to be stuck in a job that was taking away all my time from my music. It didn't make sense. My last day was the 29th of May, which was my birthday. Quitting was the perfect gift for my thirty-second year!

Now that I had time off, I could catch up on things that I needed to do. One of those things was to go for the follow-up appointment at

Moorfields Eye Hospital. I had been putting it off for too long. By the time I went, my eyes were fully back to normal, except for a slight feeling of strain.

Because I felt healthy and fine, I went to Moorfields alone this time. I did not see any reason to make William miss work. He had just started a temp job with Barclays Bank (not Citibank after all). He was paid by the hour and did not get paid for time off, so I figured it was better that he go to work.

My appointment took place in several departments. Before that day, I had no idea that so many tests were available for eyeballs. It was fascinating!

The first department I went to was called orthoptics. This is where a technician tests your vision and eye movement in hundreds of different ways. In the waiting room, I realised that many children are born with eye conditions. The night I lost my mind in the children's waiting area of A & E, I never thought about what problems children can have with their eyes.

The waiting room in this department was jam-packed with kids; some were babies. Again, as in the emergency waiting room, there were all kinds of toys for them to play with, including a big wooden rocking horse and a playhouse. The children, half of them with eyepatches, were arguing over who gets to ride the horse.

I often find children's behaviour to be impressive. They have strength that most of us lose as we get older. Forget the fact that they were arguing over the horse; that is typical of kids. All of them had been through and would probably continue to go through major procedures and tests for their eyes. Some of them had severe problems, but they did not let that stop them from their child lives. Most of them, I am sure, did not really understand why they were there exactly.

For the parents, it was a different story. Most of them looked like they had been through a lot of strain. I was thinking how difficult it must be for parents to watch their child have a medical problem and know that there is nothing they can do to completely stop it. It must be a nightmare.

I eavesdropped on some of the parents' conversations, and I learned that people came from all over England to bring their kids to this hospital. Some travelled for four or more hours by train and would then spend the night in London. I was impressed.

Inside the actual clinic, there were several testing stations set up. Each station had its own young woman in a white coat with a clipboard and a little bag filled with instruments to test and measure eyes. It was a peculiar room, I thought. Half the people in the room were covering one eye, looking at pictures, telling what they did or didn't see. Some of the kids from the waiting room were in there behaving much better than they did outside. They now had the fear of God in them. I was a little nervous as well.

I too, had my own young woman in a white coat. She was about twenty-five years old, with dark hair and warm blue eyes. She was very pretty. *All* the technicians were pretty. I wondered if it was an essential criterion to the hiring process there. They looked like actresses on a hospital soap opera.

This is an interesting job to have, I thought.

My testing began with regular eye chart tests that we have all done before. I could read the smallest line on the chart, as I always could in the past. After passing all the regular eye tests, I had to look at a picture of a little bird through different glass prisms. Some of the prisms made the bird turn into two birds. I had to keep telling the technician how many birds I saw. I apparently passed that one.

After that, she tested my eyeball movements. I would slowly move my eyes side to side and she would watch them closely with a small torch. She wanted to know how my eyes felt that day. I told her the truth, which was that they felt fine, except that they felt slightly tight.

They felt like they had been strained for a month and now they had recovered, but with small residual discomfort. She seemed satisfied with my test results. Whatever it was that caused my previous problem had obviously gone. I was sent to another department for more tests.

She sent me to the ophthalmology department. I was waiting, when yet another technician called my name to go for yet another test before I saw the ophthalmologist.

Damn, this hospital is thorough, I thought. She took me to a room to perform a test that indicates your peripheral sight. You look straight ahead inside a box and dots light up. When you see a dot, you press the button. What is great is that you get the results straight away. I did OK on this test, although one eye missed quite a few dots. The result was borderline normal, so it was no big deal.

Finally, I saw an ophthalmologist. He looked at my eyes through the scope. I really do hate those tests. The scope comes so close to the eyeballs, it makes my stomach turn. He looked behind my eyes and said everything was normal. He told me that he thought the distorted vision could have been migraine related. I thought that was an interesting theory, which was just as valid as any other reason. He told me that if it ever came back again, I would need to see a neurologist for further investigation.

Well, I was sure that it would never come back again. The important thing was that it was all over, and I was going to have a terrific summer of suntanning in the park and learning my way around this great city. Or so I thought....

Birth of the Awkward Bitch

ℬ

The summer of 2004 began fairly well. William was settling into his job with Barclays Bank, in its compliance department. He was still working as a temp, which meant that he had no yearly contract, no paid holiday time, and not a lot of job security. Despite this, it was a good job, and the project he was working on was scheduled to last for two years. He was glad to be working again and I was glad to not be working (at least in theory I was). I was still feeling a bit drained from my eye ordeal; I felt that I needed to take it easy for a while.

William and I began playing our music at open-mic nights and learning about the London music scene. Every Tuesday night, we were playing at one particular pub in Islington. As we didn't have a band yet, we played there not only to spread our music but also to meet other musicians, perhaps potential bandmates.

By day, I was suntanning in the park and trying to relax. I was also wishing I had another job lined up so that I could enjoy the time off a little more thoroughly. I needed the security.

I started to worry about running out of money, which can happen so quickly in London. I found it difficult to settle my thoughts.

I decided that I needed to see my mother. I had just been through a mysterious illness, and for the first time in my life, my mom was not physically there to comfort me. She was on the phone almost every night, but it's not the same. I was feeling homesick.

So, in the middle of June, I flew home alone. William could not get time off at his job, not that we could afford to have him take time off anyway. Seeing my family was just what I needed. I was so happy to be back in my old surroundings. The three months I had lived in London seemed like a dream.

My mom thought that I looked too skinny and a bit too tired. My sisters commented that I looked drained and run-down. One of my sisters, Lisa, who is a veterinarian, said that I looked a little malnourished. She questioned what I was eating in London and where exactly we were living. They were each definitely concerned about the youngest child.

The summer heat of New York made me feel more tired. I thought nothing of it though, because heat makes everyone feel a little sluggish at times. I was home for only six days. I did not tell any of my friends that I was back. This was partly because I looked like crap and did not want them to ask what the hell was happening to me over in London. The other and most important reason was that all I wanted to do was lie down on my mom's sofa and drink lots of tea with my sisters and her. I just wanted to feel comfort. That was exactly what I did for the entire six days. It was like being a baby back in my cot.

When I got back to England, I expected to feel fresh after my little holiday. I didn't. William spent his days working for the bank, and I spent mine taking in more sun and interviewing for various jobs. My mind was racing at all times and I started staying up very late at night. I would stare out the window and watch the neighbourhood foxes trotting around. I became infatuated with one particular fox that lived in our garden. I was so intent on watching him that it became like a stakeout. Sometimes I would not go to sleep until I saw him at least once, even if it was into the early morning hours.

I woke up late in the day and felt crappy. I was getting more and more tired that month, but I thought it was because I was worrying all the time and keeping odd hours.

I kept saying, 'I feel like shit and I cannot stop feeling like shit.' I also looked like shit. My eyes had dark circles under them and looked glassy. I looked like I needed to sleep for a month. In fact, I had downloaded pictures that I took on my trip home, and I was disturbed by them. I could not get over how terrible I looked in them. I knew I looked bad, but I didn't think I looked as bad as the pictures revealed. My skin looked grey.

I asked William, 'Do I look this shitty in person?'

'You don't look shitty,' he insisted. 'You look beautiful, like a porcelain doll.'

From early on in our relationship, he called me his 'porcelain doll'. He still does.

'You just look a little bit tired. You need to rest more.' He saw me through rose-coloured glasses.

Someone smart might have gone to the doctor, but not me. I honestly thought that the stress of our move must have been too much for me and that I just needed time to look and feel better.

It was now early July, and we realised time was wasting by. We needed to get our music projects back up and running. We continued playing the open-mic nights while we started aggressively looking for players for William's band.

This was a top priority. His music is more technically difficult to play than mine; hence, finding people to play his music has always posed a challenge. The boys we played with in New

York had not been easy to find. So, we started auditioning many guitarists and drummers.

After two weeks of heavily auditioning people, we found the right players, but as we expected, the only musicians who could play William's songs well were *paid* musicians. We now had a new expense and, once again, money started to worry me greatly. That summer a report was published that London beat Tokyo for the most expensive city in the world to live.

Yet again, I started thinking that perhaps the move was not a good one. I started second guessing everything in my life. I would tell William, 'Maybe I don't belong here. Maybe I am not meant to be here, even though my spirit feels I am meant to be here. Maybe I wouldn't think so much if I had a great job.'

'You'll find a job soon,' he said. 'You always find a job. Besides, look at all these companies who want to meet you.'

Many companies were indeed showing interest in me at that point. I went on a fair amount of interviews. One was for store manager of Burberry in Knightsbridge. On one of my Burberry interviews (there were four in total), I found myself suddenly having to pee very urgently. This is another symptom of MS, but of course, I didn't know. The gentleman interviewing me was personable and exceedingly chatty. I started sweating. I realised quickly that if I did not go to the toilet, I was going to pee in the chair.

For a moment I thought that if I interrupted him, he would think I had a problem. But I had to go. So I just said, 'I am so sorry to interrupt you, but I had so much tea today. Could I use your toilet?'

You know what? It was absolutely fine. When I came back from the toilet, I made a joke that now I could concentrate! The man laughed. I was clearly overreacting. I got the job, by the way, but turned it down.

Another job offer was on the table, with Yves Saint Laurent. I had interviewed there the same week as Burberry. The people there were a little more hip and the product was more my style. I took their offer and started working on the 20th of July.

I loved my job immediately. It was one of those things where you just connect right away. Everyone was stylish and fresh, yet seemed to know what he or she was doing. I became the accessories department manager, in the Sloane Street store, but just five weeks later, I was promoted to ladies department manager in the Old Bond Street store. It was turning out to be a great experience. I actually enjoyed the 'day job'! I met many special people whom I am still friends with. My life was making sense!

Now that I was making money again, I felt more relaxed. It was time to concentrate on other parts of my life. It was already early September (six months since we had moved) and high time to start looking for members of the Marlo Donato band. Playing my songs at open-mic nights was still going very well. People were enjoying my music. I was feeling very good about the reaction I was getting from London audiences.

We were also enjoying the rehearsals with the new Mantis and The Prayer band. The guys were pretty cool and exceptionally talented. William's music was sounding so good. We booked our first proper London gig for October at a venue in Islington!

During this time, I was feeling almost as tired as I did in the beginning of the summer. I thought it was just because I was getting used to waking up early for work again, although usually when I start a new job, I have endless amounts of excited energy.

I figured that I was also getting used to the new, rigorous rehearsal schedule that William and I had started at night.

When we lived in New York, we rehearsed in the comfort of our own apartment. In fact, we had taken out our dining room table and replaced it with a drum kit and two guitar amplifiers. Our living room was open to the dining space. The living room part had a piano, two keyboards, three guitars, two microphone stands, another amplifier, and oh yeah, last and least importantly, a beautiful sofa!

I used to rehearse in my pyjamas with a cup of tea in my hand. Now our life was very different.

We had to haul our equipment on a bus and then walk it all about half a mile to a warehouse park with poor lighting. After rehearsal, around midnight, we'd take a night bus back home. This was really tiring, especially when it rained, but we thought it was good for our musical souls. We were paying our dues.

The night of the first gig came. It was the 12th of October, 2004. I remember I felt a bit off balance on the stage that night. I don't usually get nervous at a gig, but I felt a little on edge that night. I chalked it up to the fact that it was our first gig with the London band members.

As I was playing though, the feeling was not getting better. My fingers felt awkward as they hit the piano keys. That night I also hit my mouth off the microphone several times. I felt like I was drunk, but I had not had an ounce of liquor. As a rule, I never drink before or during my stage time. I sometimes close my eyes when I perform. Usually when I open them, I am in the same spot I was when I closed them. This was not the case on this night, though. Every time I opened my eyes I was no longer near the microphone. I would try to get close to it again and smack my lip into it.

Damn girl, I thought. *Get hold of yourself. Playing a gig with blood running off your lip is not very ladylike, though it is very rock n' roll.*

Despite my swollen lip, the first performance was a success. We all had a great time. Even so, I felt a bit weird about my awkwardness.

'Did I look OK tonight?' I asked William

'Yeah,' he answered. 'You looked *hot!*'

'No, I mean did I seem *awkward* in any way? I felt a little weird. Like not balanced or something.'

'You looked great, as always,' he said. 'You sounded great too!'

I remember telling myself that for the second gig, I would be different. I would be back to my *old self*. Somehow, though, my instincts told me otherwise. I somehow felt that my *old self* was preparing to leave me.

❧

It was during the middle of October that I began noticing bruises all over me, though mostly concentrated on my legs. William noticed them before I did.

'How the hell did you get that bruise?' he kept asking, about various ones.

I would later remember knocking into a table or a wall the day before.

'You need to be more careful!' he'd say. 'What is happening to you?'

One day I gave him the answer that would continue to be my answer for the rest of my life.

'I am one awkward bitch,' I joked.

We broke into laughter.

Many years ago, one of my sisters went through what my mom called an 'awkward stage', where she fell very often and kept scraping the same knee. She was seven years old at the time. I figured I was going through a clumsy stage too; only mine came a little later.

Not only was I slamming into walls and tables, but I also started tripping on the pavement outside. It is normal for anyone to trip once in a while, but I was tripping all the time. Even sadder is that I would look back, expecting to see a crack or bump in the pavement.

I did not think that it was my fault (I would later learn that this kind of tripping is a sign of MS). In fact, I remember ringing home and telling my family that the pavement in London is uneven everywhere. I commented, 'They should really do something about the unevenness because I am tripping all through London!' What a bitch! My apologies to London.

I continued tripping along the *supposedly* uneven and poorly made pavements of London without a real bother. Well, there was one bother, I suppose. When I was tripping, I would get some sceptical looks from people around me. This was especially the case in the morning.

I could not understand why they were looking, but now I realise that most likely they thought I was drunk or hung over. I did not have time to ponder the tripping or the looks too much anyway. I had more important things to worry about.

One of them was forming the Marlo Donato band. Finding bandmates was a little harder than I had hoped. The auditioning process was slow. I kept searching, first for a guitarist. I placed ads on local Internet websites and spoke to dozens of potential guitarists. A lot of them were either creepy guys or otherwise unsuitable persons. William came to the studio with me to help audition people, but it was not going well. I felt frustrated but still had high hopes.

It was now almost the end of October, and I was getting exceptionally stressed again. Some of it was because of my lack of bandmates, but that was not the main stressful issue. Work was going very well, and so was my social life. The problem was of a different kind.

It was a presidential election year in the United States. Before I moved to England, I had not realised just how opinionated the rest of the world felt about American elections. In fact, I had not realised how opinionated they were about Americans in general. I was ignorant in that respect. That month, the only news I ever heard in England was about the American election for president. Everywhere I went; people would hear my accent and ask what I thought about it. Sometimes people at the grocery store or at the bus stop would ask if I was American. After I said yes, they would say, 'I hope you are not voting for Bush!'

People seemed to think that I was George Bush's cousin or something. They would angrily ask me about US foreign policy. This infuriated me. I thought, *I am trying to survive in London; the most expensive city in the world. I just want to enjoy myself here and not worry about US foreign policy. I don't write the fucking foreign policy, so I wish people would stop speaking to me as if I did.*

It was becoming overwhelmingly annoying. I was getting wound up to the point of boiling. I was so tired of people pointing their finger at America, and thinking that they knew Americans. I was defending America on a daily basis, sometimes on an hourly basis, and I am not exaggerating.

When I lived in the States, I complained about the American government constantly. That was when I was amongst fellow Americans, though. Whilst living in England, I certainly was not going to say anything against the land where I was born.

I was fed up. I felt like jumping on the next plane to New York. William was getting the same reactions and he was fed up too. Every night he and I had the same conversation.

I would ask, 'Did people annoy the shit out of you about the election today?'

'Yep,' he would answer. 'Yet again, I was verbally attacked. I told them off.'

We were both furious. We joked that we should start pretending that we were Canadian until after the election. As upsetting as all this was, the hoopla over the American presidential election was soon to be overshadowed by something else. The real shit was about to hit the fan.

Wonderland

&

On a rainy morning at the end of October, I woke up in *Wonderland*. I knew from the second I opened my eyes that something was terribly wrong. I could not focus properly at all. There was a blue lantern that hung from our ceiling in the bedroom with little glass beads hanging off of it. As I looked up at it, the lantern moved into two images for a second and then went back to one.

'Please God, don't let this happen to me again,' I begged out loud. I kept a small bottle of holy water on the nightstand by our bed. I immediately reached for it, rubbed some on my eye, and prayed. I thought to myself *I must be too stressed out. That's why this shit is coming back. I can't stress out over this stupid election.*

That morning I felt an exhaustion that made me want to vomit. Lifting my head from the pillow was a feat. The feeling of bubbles in my head seemed to be starting as well. I slowly got out of bed, adjusting to the weirdness that was taking over my vision. I gagged as I brushed my teeth. I felt like crying but frankly did not have the energy to squeeze out one tear. I was filled with more confusion than sadness anyway.

After several minutes, my eyes adjusted and the weirdness seemed to dissipate. I pulled myself together and shuffled off to work. I told my staff that my eyes felt a bit weird, so if they thought I was looking at them strangely, they should not think that I was crazy.

At work, I had become friends with one particular colleague called Colin. He was the same age as me. He was, and is, a lovely guy. He reminds me of a grown-up version of *The Little Prince*, with his blond hair, fair skin, and blue eyes. He is tall and fit. To this day, I have to wipe the drool off of everyone who meets him. Oddly, he was one of the only people at work who was actually English. We had an immediate rapport, where we could tell each other straight, just how it is. There was no bullshit between us.

That day, I pulled him to the side. I asked him, 'Tell me the truth. Do my eyes look fucked up? Do I look weird?'

'No weirder than usual,' he replied. He had a wicked sense of humour too. We both laughed.

'No really,' I said. 'Do I look like I am looking directly at you? Are my eyes off in any way? Please look closely.'

He stared into my eyes. 'You look fine, darling.'

I felt a little relieved, but I felt so strange that I thought I must *look* strange too. I asked more colleagues if I looked all right. Everyone insisted that I looked normal.

I had hired a new girl to start that day and all I could think was that she must think I had mad eyes. I was showing her around and introducing her to people, all the while not being able to really focus on her. It bothered me that I couldn't give her my usually thorough training.

That afternoon turned out to be OK. My vision was slightly off, but my eyes did not feel as awful as they had in the morning. I was tripping everywhere, though. I remember thinking, *Damn! The awkward bitch is back in full force! What the hell is wrong with me?* I was trying to laugh it off. The new girl saw me trip a few times. The first time she said something like 'be careful.' The next couple of times she just gave a little sympathetic smile.

Hours passed. As evening approached, my condition stopped getting better. In fact, around 4 p.m., it started getting worse again. I began feeling an intense pressure in my eyeballs. With that, my vision also decreased. The world looked more and more out of focus. I slowly realised that everything was doubling slightly like the lantern had that morning.

Every display showcase in our shop had small light bulbs that ran on a track. There were literally hundreds of these little lights throughout the shop. All of the lights seemed to smear in different directions. It was like in the film *Star Wars*, when spaceships go into hyperspace! Watching the 'hyperspace' lights while trying to conduct my daily business was very distracting. Added to that was the fact that a blind spot emerged on the right side. Suddenly, when I looked to the right, there was darkness. Now distraction and annoyance turned to terror in a space of twenty minutes.

I also started to lose my balance completely, and I fell down on a staircase. I pulled the muscles in my arm trying to hold onto the banister, stopping the fall.

A couple of people asked me if I had been partying.

Fantastic, I thought. *I look like a druggie.* Colin suddenly seemed worried. He was no longer making jokes with me.

'You have gone a bit pale now,' he said. 'Maybe you should go home early.'

I kept laughing and saying, 'No, really, I am totally fine.' I did not want to leave early. I felt that if I went home early then I would have to admit something was wrong, and I was not ready for that. I was still in denial. *This weirdness cannot be happening again,* I thought. *I won't let it. I'll stop it.*

When I returned home that evening, I got straight into bed. I felt weak. The tiredness and strange feelings were overwhelming.

'I'm taking you to the hospital,' William said.

'I can't go the hospital. I'm too tired,' I said. 'I think I'm just stressed out lately. I'll be fine once I just rest.'

William did not agree. 'Maybe, I should call an ambulance, Marlo.'

'No way,' I said. 'I'm OK. I just need to sleep.'

'I don't like this,' he said. 'You are *not* OK! If you are not better tomorrow, you cannot go to work! You are so stubborn! This is bullshit!'

The next morning, I woke up in worse condition. My vision was more distorted and the strange feelings in my head and eyes were more prevalent. The blind spot to the right was slightly bigger. I did the same routine as the day before, gagging my way through brushing my teeth. I told William that I felt much better but would probably stay home in bed. This white lie helped me get my way. William went to work and did not try to persuade me to see a doctor or go to hospital.

'Make sure you rest in the bed and don't go food shopping or anything,' he said as he kissed me goodbye. 'I'll bring home a dinner for us.'

'OK,' I lied.

I stupidly went to work again! I don't like missing work, especially for what I consider dumb reasons. Stress was a poor reason to miss work. This was all surely stress related. I would just have to pull myself together and be strong.

Believe it or not, I continued going to work for several days like that! By the sixth or seventh day, I could function only by closing one eye. I was tripping throughout the shop. I could not walk 100 yards without tripping. I also could not walk a straight line outdoors. On my lunch break, I was walking at angles down the street. I would start off walking near the curb and, moments later, I would sway towards the buildings and sometimes brush off the walls.

Indoors, I felt like I was on an obstacle course from hell.

'Ooh! Ouch! Oh! Whew!' I said all day as I bumped into chairs, tables, and walls. Basically, I looked like a drunk with a growing bruise count.

I also bumped into customers, which was embarrassing. One day, I knocked into a customer's handbag, which went flying up in the air. It didn't fall, as it was strapped to her shoulder, but *I* almost fell.

'Oops!' I said. 'I beg your pardon, Madam.' She was unimpressed by my actions and gave me the 'mind where you're going' icy glare.

At that point, I did not think the day could get any worse, so of course it did. Sometime after lunch, I started hallucinating. Oh yes, this is when the real fun began.

In actual fact, it was not fun at all. I was at the till, and as I was looking at the computer screen, I saw a pen from the desk lift off into the air! It was in my peripheral view. It lifted off in a slow, anticlockwise motion. It made a little circle in the air.

What the hell? I thought. But as I turned to look at it, the pen was back on the desk, where it should be. *OK*, I thought. *What the fuck was that about? What just happened to me?* I was utterly confused.

When I turned to look back at the computer screen, the pen was in the air again, moving ever so slowly. It made the same little circular journey that it did before. I took a dramatic step back from the till.

'OK!' I said to one of my colleagues. 'I need to tell you that I am now hallucinating! I am going to remain calm, but I just saw that pen floating in the air! I am fucking hallucinating!'

'Girl, you are lucky!' he said smiling. 'You didn't take anything?'

'No!' I said. 'I am hallucinating for no reason!'

'Enjoy it!' he said with a straight face. 'Do you know what I would have to take to get to that point? And how much I would have to pay? Honey, you are getting it for *free!*'

We burst into laughter. It was yet another moment from *Marlo's surreal world* and although the situation was alarming, to say the least, I laughed it off and continued working as if nothing had happened. The truth was, though, that my colleagues were a bit concerned about the hallucination incident. They were already bewildered by my behaviour during the previous week. I can't imagine what they must have thought my problem was.

Colin asked me to come into his office.

'Enough is enough,' he said to me. 'You better go to the doctor.' I knew that he was right. None of this was even close to normal. I was clearly unwell. I decided I would go home, have dinner, and maybe visit the eye hospital again.

So, after work, I headed for my usual train. My commute was always the same: I would take the tube from Green Park to Stockwell and then change for the Northern line to Clapham Common. That night, there was extra commotion on the trains. It was Guy Falkes Day, or Bonfire Night, as it is also known as.

For those who don't know what this is, I'll briefly explain. Guy Falkes was a mercenary who was part of a plot to burn down the Houses of Parliament back in the year 1605. He was caught, tortured, and sentenced to death. The king at the time (James I) declared the 5th of November as a national holiday so that people would not forget what happened and celebrate that he (the king) was not killed! To this day, fireworks are displayed and bonfires are lit on this night. People in London really get into it! (Which still baffles William and me, but that's beside the point!)

Needless to say, people were going out in droves. Fires were set in celebration throughout the city. (Some were legal, many were not!) People were out drinking and screaming. It was chaotic, especially for me, considering the state I was in.

Because of 'fires and police activity', as the station announcements told us, the Northern line trains stopped running for a while. There were so many people at Stockwell station that I could not navigate through them. My eyesight suddenly got much worse. In an instant I could not see clearly in any direction. Everything was smearing into two. It was like looking at two negative images on top of one another again, except this time, you had taken LSD as well! It was worsened by the fact that there were so many people and they were moving so fast. I was pushed and shoved in every direction. It was hard to keep my balance and not fall. I couldn't see the ground. I couldn't focus my eyes on anything. It was like my eyes just stopped working entirely.

I was walking with my hands in front of me. I was stumbling, and I was afraid that I would fall onto the tracks. Even worse was the fear that I would not only fall onto the tracks but would accidentally push someone as well.

People most likely assumed that I was drunk. In a way, I was hoping that they did think that. That would be more normal than what was really happening, whatever it was.

I wanted to stop and start screaming, 'EVERYONE, PLEASE STOP MOVING!' I thought about grabbing someone and saying, 'Please help me!' I couldn't stop, though. I kept walking, trying to keep up with the massive crowds.

The tube staff continued making announcements about the police activity and suggested that passengers should make their way outside and get bus service. I did not know that area of town yet, except that it had a bad reputation. I figured I should take their advice or I would never get home.

I was so tired. All I wanted was to get home and rest for a few minutes before going to hospital. I longed for my bed. I stumbled up the steps, making my way towards the exit of the station. I clutched the banister and then the wall. I was almost crawling at one point, and yet no one offered me assistance. Everyone was too busy pushing and running in different directions.

It was a colossal struggle for me. It was dark outside, and the street was heavily lit. Everything looked distorted in my eyes. The streetlights were melting into one another. The lights of cars were smeared into each other as well. I could not see anything clearly. It was like a nightmare from which I would never wake up. I tried to look across the street, which was like looking into an abstract painting whose creator painted it in drug rehab. There was no way I could cross it. The street itself may as well have been water, because I couldn't see it.

I did not even know which direction I lived in. I didn't know which side of the street I should take the bus and I could not see another person clearly enough to ask directions.

As I stood there looking both ways over and over, I became very confused as to where I was altogether. I don't mean what *street* I was on. I mean what *city* I was in. I felt like I didn't know who I was, actually. I felt detached from my own body. I tried closing one eye and walking.

I went over to rest against a fence and ring William. I could barely push the buttons on the phone. I had to keep one eye closed and hold the phone up in the air and to the left. That was the only angle where I could see the phone. I must have looked like I was on drugs at that moment. I was desperate. There was no answer at home. William was not home yet, probably because of the delays.

I tried to hold back the tears, but I couldn't. I started sobbing uncontrollably. I couldn't believe the situation I was in. I have never been so scared in my life. I was utterly confused and desperate.

What is happening to me? The thought was deafening in my mind. I felt like I was being tortured. I started to wonder if it was real. *Maybe I am having a bad dream.* I put my hands up to my face, crying there in front of every passer-by. I started to think that I had a brain tumour and that I would die on the street. This seemed to be the most logical explanation. *I am dying. I am dying alone in a city, where no one even knows who I am. I have a paper in my bag that has my name on it. The police will find it and they will be able to trace William.*

I thought of what happened to me at Canary Wharf. *I lived through that. This is not the same, though. I will not live through this.* The whole scenario was so much more intense than what happened to me at Canary Wharf. There, the thought had also occurred to me that I might die in the street, but this time, I was more certain. In a way, I wanted to die. I wanted anything that would take me away from the nightmare that was my reality. It was a living hell.

Then, in a single instant, the paralysing fear that was encompassing me left like a bolt of lightning. It was replaced by a wave of anger that swept through me.

Fuck this, I thought. *I am not dying here! I did not come to London to fucking die! I am not dying like this! I fucking refuse!*

I wiped my tears and forced myself to get away from the fence. I stumbled back down to the tube station and waited against a wall. The trains started running again, but I could not get on. There were too many people and I could not steer through them. People were still pushing each other like cattle. At first, I did not dare try to move from the wall. As the crowds went from chaotic to slightly overcrowded, I found a seat in the station. I sat there while train after train went by. I waited until there were no more crowds of people. I sat there for over two hours, just staring straight ahead at my messed-up world.

When the station finally cleared, I got on a deserted train. Talking to myself mentally, I made my way back home. *You can do it. One hundred more steps, fifty more steps, a few more steps. You're almost there.*

When I got home, William was just getting in the door as well. When he turned around saying hello, I heard the happy music of his voice turn to horror. He could see straight away that I was not well.

'We're going to the hospital *now*,' he said sternly.

'I know,' I said and started crying again.

'You're going to be all right. I am with you and I am not going to let anything happen to you,' he said, picking me up in his arms.

We immediately went to Moorfields Eye Hospital.

Is It a Tumour?

so

In the waiting room in A & E, I held onto William, desks and chairs for balance. My severely distorted world seemed to continue its downward spiral. Every time I thought I reached a plateau, things would get just a little bit worse. Everything I looked at was moving in and out of itself. It was nauseating.

At one point, I became fixated on one particular object in the waiting room. There was a registration desk with a giant plant on it. To me, it looked like there were two desks and two giant plants. One of the desks was on roller skates and would roll away from the other one and then roll back into it. Each time it rolled back, the desk would almost become one object. But just as this happened, the second desk would roll away again.

The desks would roll as far apart as half the room. I told William to look over at the registration desk as I described to him what I saw and how I was figuring out which desk was the real one.

I explained to him, 'At first, it's hard to tell what objects are real and what images are their doubles. I realise now, looking at this desk, all objects to the left of the doubles are the real thing. The right one is the double. Jesus Christ, it's amazing.'

That was a great discovery, because from then on, I could tell which objects were really there. You don't want to sit on a chair that is the double and fall on your bum!

All kinds of dread began to sweep over me as we sat in that waiting room. I suppose it was the fear of all the things I had been thinking in secret for the past week.

I kept asking William, 'Do you think I have a brain tumour?'

'No. You don't have a brain tumour. If it was a brain tumour then you never would have gotten better the first time.' He squeezed my hand reassuringly.

'Then what do I have?' I asked.

'I don't know,' he said. 'But it's not a brain tumour.'

Minutes passed. 'How do you know it's not a brain tumour, William?'

'I just know. Now try to clear your mind of these kinds of thoughts.'

I was silent for a few minutes again. Then I asked, 'Are you *sure* it's not a brain tumour?' I asked him so many times, I'm sure he was mentally drained. We both agreed that it was not a virus or a migraine. But what was it? We felt like we were in something inescapable. We were.

The doctor who saw me that night was a very clever lady. There are some doctors who are so gentle yet confident that they immediately put you at ease. She was like that. I knew I was in good hands. She examined me thoroughly, saying that the muscle of my right eye was slightly paralysed, though the effect was subtle. When she asked me to move my eyes to the right, one eyeball did not move all the way. Neither William nor I had noticed this until she pointed it out. When you looked at me closely, one eye would turn into my nose, and the other could not turn as far. It looked terrible when you realised it. No wonder I felt so much pressure on my eyeball!

She told me that I would need to see a neurologist, but first she wanted blood work drawn up. She gave me a prescription for blood tests, but as it was Friday night, the lab was closed. She commented that she also wanted another colleague to look at my eye, but he wouldn't be there until Monday. William and I would have to wait until then.

I left the hospital that night with a large cotton wool eyepatch taped on my face. This turned out to be quite useful in a number of ways. The first was that it was much easier to see with one eye constantly covered. Another was that everyone on the tube gets out of your way because they *see* you have a problem. Another still, is that you don't look as dumb when you are off balance. People assume that you have an eye injury that has caused you to lose your balance. Now people wouldn't look at me suspiciously when I tripped. It made me feel better.

When we got home, William took out the blood test prescription that the doctor had written out.

'She wrote something weird on this,' he said. 'Diplopia, possible Nerve VI Palsy, cause?'

'What does that mean?' I asked. 'Palsy? I have palsy? Oh my God!'

'People are *born* with cerebral palsy,' William said. 'You don't have palsy.'

'Then what did she write?' I asked.

I immediately started looking it up on the Internet. I was in no condition to be Internet surfing, and William was pleading with me to log off the computer and go to bed.

'I can't go to bed after someone writes that I might have some kind of palsy!' I said. I was overtired at that point. I felt completely shattered. With the patch still over my eye, I strained to see the damn computer screen, but I had to know what this problem was. The word *palsy* sounded so bad. All I could think of was brain damage.

I learned that all the word *palsy* means is *paralysis*.

'I have a paralysis of the sixth cranial nerve,' I triumphantly announced to William. *Great*, I thought. *Solved. Wait a minute. What the hell does that mean?*

What I learned was this; there are twelve nerves that come from our brain stem. They are called *cranial nerves*. Any one of them can become dysfunctional for any number of reasons. The sixth nerve affects movement of the eyes, which then affects vision. When this nerve is paralysed, it causes *diplopia*, which is a fancy word for *double vision*. Even more specific, it causes side-by-side double vision, which is what I experienced.

As I read more and more, I knew that this was what I had. What a relief! Sort of. But what was the cause?

The websites listed all the possible causes of nerve VI palsy. They were from mild to very serious. One cause was multiple sclerosis, and another cause was a type of tumour. Now the tumour thoughts were back in force. I started to panic inside. I felt my heart sinking. I kept thinking that my family would be scarred forever if this were the case. The youngest child of the family moved to London only to die a few months later from an inoperable brain tumour.

I got into bed but couldn't fall asleep. Too many thoughts were tormenting my mind. William put a film on for me to fall asleep to. It was *Shrek*. I had taken my eyepatch off in bed.

'Does this movie have two donkeys in it?' I asked. I tried to laugh.

'No, just one donkey,' William answered. 'Try to relax and close your eyes,' he said, caressing me.

'Do I have a brain tumour?' I asked for the hundredth time that night.

William turned to me very seriously and took my head in his great big hands. He closed his eyes. He was performing a kind of 'visualization' that we would do for each other if one of us had a headache. We try to visualize where the pain is and remove it.

We fell silent for several minutes, as he gently touched different parts of my head.

'You don't have a tumour,' he said. 'But you have something on or in your brain, Marlo. I see something: a shadow.' He then told me that he visually sent a 'shark' in to get whatever it was out. 'The shark can't get it all,' he said, pulling me closer. We fell asleep in a tight cuddle.

Early Monday morning, we were back at Moorfields Eye Hospital. I saw the doctor whom the previous lady doctor had recommended. He examined me and agreed that it was probably nerve VI palsy, and that they would need to look deeper for a cause. He sent me down another corridor to the lab for blood tests. This was a quick visit, which took less than ten minutes. I started to feel like a car on an assembly line, going from one stop to another. I knew from my previous visit that there were many departments and that the staff members in each knew what they were doing.

The doctor came back and brought me down another corridor. We walked into another department: neuro-ophthalmology. He told us that they usually don't take people without appointments, but they were going to fit me in. This made me nervous. Getting 'fit in' to see a hairdresser is a good thing. Getting 'fit in' to see a brain specialist is not.

I was obviously brought here because I have a major brain problem. They are going to tell me that I have a brain tumour, but they will need a scan to make sure. Calm down, Marlo, it could be anything. This was my internal dialogue for the entire two hours we sat waiting in that department. At one point, my internal dialogue started talking so fast that I thought it was speaking in tongues. I wanted to jump up screaming, 'Shut up! Just shut the fuck up!'

It was only interrupted by external dialogue with William that was much along the same lines. I think William said, 'You don't have a tumour' at least ten times.

'I do. I have a tumour,' I kept saying. 'I do.'

Sitting there was torment for us. He denies it to this day, but I know it was very hard for him to sit in that room and pretend that things would be OK. He had a lot of hope, though: more than I did.

In the neuro-ophthalmology clinic, three doctors examined me, one by one. I was asked a complete history of my health.

'Did you ever have a head injury?' the first one asked me. He was a very young man.

'Yes!' I answered. 'I had a concussion last year when I accidentally smashed my head on a brick while standing up in my garden. It was a bizarre accident. Could that be the reason for these problems?'

'It's doubtful,' he said, looking down at his clipboard. 'Have you ever had migraine headaches?'

'Yes,' I said. 'I had them a very long time ago. They would come on every three or four months. They would start in the early morning and last until the late afternoon. I haven't had them for a long time, though.'

As I spoke about the migraines, he was busy jotting everything down on his clipboard. He started jotting so much that I was no longer sure if he was hearing every word I said. William and I were getting a bit frustrated with him.

At this point a second doctor came over and started looking at the notes the first doctor was writing down. The two of them chatted to each other about my history and would then turn back to me to ask another question. Then they chatted again and looked back to me again.

I started to feel very uneasy. *Where are they going with these questions?*

Finally, the first doctor concluded that I did have nerve VI palsy (now all the doctors agreed). He told us that he thought my problems were probably migraine related. I asked him if it was normal for migraines to last days, or weeks like it did in April. I had never heard of such a thing. He said it could happen.

I was not convinced. In fact, I started to resent him. I quickly realised that the only thing worse than a terrible diagnosis is no diagnosis, or a bullshit diagnosis. I couldn't go home in this condition and accept that this was a type of migraine. My gut instinct told me he was wrong. He was looking for a quick solution at my expense. I felt like screaming, 'This is no fucking migraine!'

He told me that we could do an MRI (brain scan), but it probably wasn't necessary. He wanted to ask his superior, though, so he and the second doctor went out to get him.

'Is he crazy?' William whispered. 'Who has ever heard of a migraine lasting *this* long? He is just looking for an easy diagnosis. He should just do an MRI.'

I agreed.

The doctor brought over his superior. This one was a Mister. (A Mister, if you don't know, is a surgeon who has been accepted in the Royal

Surgical Colleges.) The Mister examined me and looked at my history.

'How long have you lived here?' he asked.

'Several months,' I replied.

'Are you being treated for something in the States?' he asked, almost suspiciously.

'No.'

I started thinking that he thought I had a tumour and came to England to have it removed for free under socialised medicine. He must have thought that I had no insurance when I lived in the States. Little did he know that I had excellent health insurance when I lived there. He looked as if he suspected what was wrong with me, as he asked me about other parts of my body, including my hands and feet.

'Any tingling or numbness anywhere?' he asked.

I told him about the numbness in my toe. Throughout the duration of his questions, I started to remember that I had tingling sensations in my fingers at certain times, but I thought that was just from sleeping on them. Doesn't everyone get that? I wasn't sure if I should bother mentioning it, but finally I did.

He looked at the young doctor and said, 'Order an urgent MRI.'

I felt like fainting. I felt like I was about to be handed a death sentence. I was very confused. Ten minutes ago I was angry because the young doctor did not want to order an MRI, and now I was freaking out because the Mister wanted me to have an urgent one. Maybe it was just the word 'urgent'.

William looked like I felt. He nervously started asking the Mister what it could be, but the Mister was aloof! He did not want to alarm us, I suppose.

He said, 'Let's just see. Now remember,' he added. 'An urgent MRI in England is not the same as an urgent MRI in the United States. You will have to wait about two weeks. Otherwise, though, you would have to wait several months.'

This made me feel better. Obviously, if it were a tumour, I would be admitted to a hospital straight away. Surely they would do an MRI that day, so that I would have enough time to make arrangements for my funeral.

I asked him, 'What if in two weeks, whatever is wrong with my brain heals? Maybe nothing will show up then?'

His answer said it all. 'Two weeks won't make a difference. The MRI will have the answers.'

In my opinion, this meant that he was looking for something specific. He knew exactly what he was looking for, but he was not telling us. *Is this because he is a British doctor? Maybe it's just their way. They give little information and come across a bit cold. Am I reading too much into it? What the hell is going on?*

We left that department knowing that I definitely had a paralysis of the sixth cranial nerve, and an MRI would probably show us why. But our day at Moorfields was still not over.

Next, we went to the orthoptics department (the one with all the pretty ladies in white coats). Looking at the rocking horse again (which now looked like two rocking horses), I could not believe that I was back there. William was shocked by how many kids were there. I explained to him that this was the department where they perform many visual tests on your eyes. I told him that the technicians were all young and very pretty, so for him, waiting there would be painless!

That day I met the most incredible technician of the bunch. Her name was Despina. She conducted many tests, which I performed horribly on. It was embarrassing. The last time I took the tests, I had done so well. Now, I was failing every single one. My eyes were like someone else's. I could not control all the bad things that were happening. It made me very sad.

Despina took me into a room that had a big board divided in the centre by a mirror that was perpendicular to it. I had to sit with my nose against the edge of the mirror. Each side of my face had a mirror reflection on it. I started to think that I would have been more comfortable taking a driver's test instead. Despina turned down the lights in the room and gave me a pointer stick. She then turned on the board. It was lighted with a grid on it that had dots. I had to point to each dot. I thought I was doing incredibly well because I could see all the dots. Then I heard William let out a small gasp.

'Oh my God,' he whispered under his breath.

What is he on about? I thought. 'Aren't I doing well?' I asked.

'Keep focusing on the screen,' Despina said softly. 'Do not worry.'

What was happening was that I was seeing the dots in a different place from where they really were. Each time I thought I pointed to a dot, I was pointing to a space that was about 6 inches from the dot.

Despina tested each eye, and it became clear that my right eye was much worse than the left.

The final test was also astonishing. It was the bird test that I had done months before. Despina had me look at the picture of the little bird, which of course I saw two of, without looking through a prism. Then she had me look at the bird through the different prisms. As the prisms got stronger, the double of the bird got closer to the original! Finally, after looking through about five prisms, the birds became one. I could see normally! It was incredible! It was like magic. I was amazed. I felt pure happiness over something so simple. She said she would stick a prism on a pair of glasses, and that is how I would see for the next few weeks.

The only problem was that I did not wear glasses. I would need to get a pair of clear glasses, so she brought me to the next department: specs.

In the specs department, I had to pick out a pair of frames, which they would fit with clear glass. The technician there showed me the five styles that were available free of charge. They looked insane.

'Oh my God,' I said as I tried on a roundish pair. '*Harry Potter* goes to hell.'

She giggled. 'Our adult patients are usually much older than you,' she said. 'They are not very stylish.'

That was an understatement. Just because people are old does not mean that they can't be stylish. When she got up to get another tray of glasses, I whispered to William, 'These glasses are not suitable for a corpse! I wouldn't be caught dead in these!'

I looked over at a carousel with many beautiful frames on it, but they were astronomically expensive. Unfortunately, we did not have much money at the time, so we were forced to look at the tray of cheap specs the girl brought over. They were a step up from the five terrible ones.

I found a pair that William thought I looked decent in. They looked OK, but were still a bit granny-ish. I did not feel good in them, but what the hell. I was so tired; I just wanted to get home to bed.

When the glasses were ready, I was sent back to see Despina in the orthoptics department. Despina attached a plastic stick-on prism over the right lens. It's called a Fresnel prism, by the way, and it's the best invention since sliced bread. As soon as I put the glasses on, all the doubling stopped! The stick-on prism was the same strength of the prism that I had looked through earlier that day in the bird test. Her instructions were to only look straight ahead when wearing the specs.

'If you look to the sides, your vision will distort,' she warned.

Of course, I immediately looked to the side, and things became distorted. I laughed. 'Whoa! I see what you mean!' Then I got nauseous. 'I will only look straight ahead,' I agreed.

Despina, William, and I were all happy with my new vision. In a way, I felt like I was cured. At least now I could see in front of me. I asked her if she also had an eyepatch she could give me: a *Zorro*-type patch. This way, when I got tired of the specs, I could switch to a patch. I was thinking in my mind that a patch would look cooler than the glasses. I remembered a television advertisement we used to have in the States for one of the cosmetic lines. The model in it was wearing a black eyepatch as she graciously stepped out of a limousine. *Hmm,* I thought deviously. *I could wear the patch with dark red lipstick and slick my hair back. Yes, this could work. It could be my look for winter.*

The thought of not looking chic and fashionable was unbearable and I wouldn't allow that to happen.

She gave me a standard black eyepatch and smiled knowingly. She understood my reasons for wanting the patch. I think she thought the glasses looked better, though.

William and I left orthoptics and made our way to the cosy cafeteria at Moorfields. I knew from my previous visit that they make a very decent jacket potato there, and that was what I wanted. We were famished after this whole ordeal and we needed something comforting.

I became acquainted with my new specs whilst waiting on the queue for my potato. It was hard not to look to the sides. I quickly realised that I could not look up or down either. The countertop looked like it was on an angle. It actually looked like it might fall down. It was very disturbing. I was so busy looking down at the countertop that I did not hear the person behind the counter when she called for the next customer in the queue. Neither did I see her. The countertop enthralled me.

'Next!' she angrily screamed at me. William nudged me along. *What a damn bitch*, I thought. *I would like to see how you function in this condition. Just because I look normal, does not mean that I am OK!* I wanted to jump over the counter and smack her, but I ordered the spud instead.

We were in the hospital that day from 8 a.m. until 5 p.m. We felt like we had worked the day there. We joked that they should send us a payslip. As we left, I told William, 'When I said I wanted to see every inch of London, I did not mean the hospitals!'

Paris

During the following week, my eye problems would not let up. I was adjusting to the prism with robotic head and shoulder movements. Even though the Fresnel prism is indeed the best invention since sliced bread, it does take getting used to. There were many times when I would be out walking and feel like the pavement was actually at my waist instead of under my feet. It felt like I was walking on my hips sometimes. I would then start to feel a little nauseated.

I would switch to the patch quite often, especially at work or a music rehearsal. It was easier to play the keyboard with the patch, or just close my eyes altogether. I continued doing other normal activities such as holding store meetings. The staff got used to seeing the patch, to the point where I don't think many people noticed it anymore.

One morning, I conducted an hour-long training with the whole store. Early that morning I was not feeling well at all, and it took a great deal of willpower to get to work. I got there early and prepared my training. I was proud of myself for trying to continue business as usual. Sometimes, during these meetings, some members of the staff can get a little overzealous and speak out of turn. Within the first ten minutes of my meeting, a saleswoman blurted out that she was very tired and did not like coming in early for these meetings.

When I heard this, my blood went to a straight boil. I looked at her and said in a very loud and pissed-off tone, 'If I can get my ass in here early in this condition and conduct this meeting with this freaking eyepatch, then you have no excuse!'

There was silence. Everyone was quiet with soft smiles on their faces.

'I am sorry,' she said, and after another brief pause, I continued the meeting.

Afterwards, I started to apologise to my boss, Simon, for using inappropriate language at the meeting. He laughed.

'I loved it!' he said. 'You should show this side of you more often!'

We both laughed.

I did not want to become too much of a bitchy person. My eyes were constantly in pain and I was starting to feel overtired all the time. This can make a person very cranky. I was getting so tired during those days that I was constantly nauseated. I would sometimes go to the toilet and just gag for no reason other than exhaustion. I was exhausted enough to fall sound asleep in my chair at lunch and not hear people crashing plates and cups around.

Each morning I would close my eyes while standing up on the train. I could almost doze off while holding on to the rail. Coming out of Green Park tube station, I got into the habit of counting the steps to the street, which helped me get up them. Mayfair has a number of homeless people who sleep in doorways, and as I walked to work each morning, I would look at them and think about curling up next to them. I had no energy at all.

I was scheduled to take a business trip to Paris in a few days. This was to be my first time there. I knew that I did not feel well enough to go. In fact, I felt like dropping dead on the floor. So do you think I cancelled it? No way. I had looked forward to that trip for months, and I was going to go if it killed me.

Most girls dream of their first trip to Paris as a romantic experience with their boyfriend or husband, strolling down the Champs-Elysées. My first trip there was spent guided by two gay men, whilst I stumbled down the Champs-Elysées, wearing the eyepatch.

I arrived at Waterloo station, wearing my granny glasses à la stick-on prism. I was going to meet Colin and Simon on the train. We were leaving a day early so that we could sightsee. This day happened to be the tenth anniversary of the Eurostar train. There were all kinds of celebrations in the station, including a rock band, clowns, and stilt walkers. The noise level was high. Music was blasting and it was very crowded. I employed my new procedure of pre-navigation: find a wall to stand near and assess the situation.

I took in the scenery at Waterloo: mostly just a sea of people. I found what would be my safest path through the sea. I revved myself up like a car does before the flags go down on the raceway. Trying to navigate through the crowds was a task. I was terrified that I would knock into one of the stilt walkers. Even worse, I noticed that there was a man filming the whole thing with a television camera. Imagine if my awkwardness was caught on film? I would be mortified. People watching their television would think, 'Look at that drunken slut, wobbling around at 8 a.m. She's probably coming down after a night of binge drinking.' Knowing my luck, I was sure to be filmed.

I did my new walk, which includes a technique of looking dead straight ahead, with my hands slightly out. A woman stopped me in my tracks and asked for directions somewhere.

'I can't fucking see,' I wanted to say. Again, no matter where I am, people stop me for directions. In the condition I was in, I found it hilarious. To my amazement, she was oblivious to my prism. She was so sweet, I would have felt bad saying that I could not see where the hell I was going, never mind tell her where to go. So, I did my usual; I closed one eye and made myself strain to see my surroundings. I was able to direct her, and this made me feel good. I laughed inside as she thanked me and went on her way. I wanted to thank her. It was a small victory.

I got on the train, which was another small task because there was a bloody big gap between the platform and the train. I saw Simon was already in his seat. As soon as I saw him I started laughing. Because of the stressful journey and the lady asking me for directions, I had been dying to laugh for the past hour. It is hard to burst into laughter when you are alone, especially when you are stumbling. Colin jumped onto the train just as the train doors were shutting. He was clearly hung over from the night before.

'Jesus, look at the state of you,' I said, as he sprawled into his seat.

We all laughed.

Riding in an aboveground train was difficult in my condition. I could not look out the window at the countryside because it was so distorted. I also could not look at Colin and Simon, because I could see the distortion out of the window in my peripheral view. Cows, sheep, and lamp posts all seemed to come at me so fast and blurred. It was sickening.

I couldn't help but think what a shame it was that I couldn't view the beautiful countryside. I was already planning another trip in my head. I would have to come back with William when I could see properly.

I was in the middle of a conversation with the guys when I just closed my eyes. I did not want to seem rude, but I could not stand having the distorted landscape in my peripheral view and four faces instead of two in my front view. It was overwhelming.

'Keep talking,' I said to them. 'I am not asleep. I just can't look at you right now.' I started cracking up laughing. 'Look at the state of me!'

They laughed.

'Don't laugh too hard, Colin. I'm in better shape than you today!'

'Yes darling, you are,' he agreed.

We continued our conversation and laughed most of the way to Paris.

When I arrived in my hotel room later that afternoon, I was exhausted. I felt a kind of tiredness that must come after staying awake for days. I looked at the bed, wanting to collapse on it so badly. I had told the guys a few minutes earlier that I wanted to sightsee with them. I proceeded to have an argument with myself. *Sick Marlo* said, 'You are too tired to go, and you need your rest.' *Fun Marlo* said, 'Are you crazy? You did not come to Paris a day early to sleep! You better pull yourself together, and get your ass out there! Paris is waiting, bitch!' I don't know how I did it, but I listened to *Fun Marlo.*

Colin, Simon, and I walked around the city for ages. We wandered through interesting little shops and courtyards. I had no idea where we were going. I just let them lead. I was so happy to be there. Paris was the most beautiful city I had ever seen, or seen two of, as was the case with me. I was wearing the granny glasses still. Colin helped me cross the streets, holding me by the arm and saying, 'Come on, Auntie!' It was comical. Every time I stopped to think of how crazy this scenario was, I would laugh. I joked about how nice it was to see both Eiffel Towers. The laughter kept me sane and helped me take my mind off the terrible pain I felt behind my eyes.

I decided that the glasses were not chic enough, though, and that I would switch to my *Zorro* patch. Again I thought of the cosmetics advertisement.

'How do I look, Colin?' I asked.

'Fabulous, darling! The patch will be all the rage next season.'

I smiled at the thought.

'You're a trendsetter,' Simon added.

We walked the entire day! I had a wonderful time. I forgot how tired I was until I got back to my room. I had been in various stages of pain all day. Night-time was usually the worst time for pain, and that night was no exception. The pain in my eyes was becoming unbearable. That dull, yet insanely intense ache was setting in for the night, like an evil little bedtime companion.

I had over-the-counter drugs from England, the United States, and France. Nothing even took the edge off of the pain. At times like this, I used to think, *This is why some people start taking major illegal drugs.* Class A drugs suddenly can look very appealing.

Pain can make you weak. I admit that, at times, pain made me feel desperate. I felt that if someone offered me heroin, or better yet, opium, I would thank him or her and take it. Those were just fantasies, though. Reality was I would try to mentally block out the pain. So, instead of trying to comb the Parisian streets for drug dealers, I decided to lie down.

I could barely get in my pyjamas. The room was spinning. I put on the television and literally fell into the bed. I listened to the news. It was soothing to hear the news in French: so melodic. It was surreal. My mind wandered. *I am half blind. I am exhausted and dizzy. I am ill. I am alone. Shit, I am in Paris. I love Paris. I love the French language. News is much better in French! Vive La France!*

I stubbornly wanted to watch the news, not just listen to it. I put a pillow over one eye and tried to watch a little bit. I flicked through other channels and stopped on the BBC because something caught my attention.

I saw something that night that I could not even make up if I tried. They were reporting on the celebration of' Eurostar's tenth anniversary. I saw a girl on TV, wearing a scarf that was identical to the one I had worn that morning. It was quite unusual. It was an oriental black-and-red satin and velvet scarf. Of course, it was not someone else. The scarf was mine! The girl was me! The irony was overwhelming. I had long dreamed of being on television, but certainly not like this. Earlier that morning I hoped I would not be caught on camera and there I was, standing like a desperado in my granny glasses for the entire world to see. 'For God's sake,' I whispered to myself. 'This is how I make my debut in France! What the fuck?' My last sleepy thought was, *Pourquoi?* I fell into a coma-like sleep.

The next day was one of the toughest days I have ever had in my life. I knew I had a gruelling day of meetings ahead of me. Even before this crap happened to me, my colleagues had told me that the meetings in Paris were long and draining. They warned me that with the combination of the rooms not having air, and being given too much information, everyone starts to fall asleep. What makes the sleepiness worse is that there are two translators in the back of the room, who translate the meetings through headsets that all the non-French-speakers wear.

My French bosses were aware of my struggle that day. They told me if I needed to leave at any time, they would get me a cab back to the hotel. I thought that was very kind of them, though I had no intention of missing any part of it. I felt that I could not let my condition stop me.

During the first meeting, I did experiments with my eyes: glasses on, glasses off. Look quickly to the left, look slowly to the right. I was in a fairly big showroom, with chairs set up in about thirty rows. I was sitting towards the back and figured no one would notice my behaviour, whilst they directed their attention towards the front of the room. I had been conducting these self-experiments for about an hour, when I realised that one of our top bosses was staring at me. She was one of those bosses who scare people without meaning to. She had a coldness about her, although I'm sure she was a very nice person really. She was always dressed in neutral colours, and she often wore something in leather. Her glares were scary. She looked at people like she was looking inside them, with her eyes partially squinted. She must have thought I was insane at that moment. I scrapped the glasses and put on the patch at one point. I saw her watching me do that too. Her face was comical, actually. Her usual squint was *squintier* than ever! Who knows what she was thinking. She looked baffled, though, that's for sure.

I continued the experiments whilst my buyer was giving a presentation. I removed my headphones from one ear, so that I could hear his sexy voice. I removed the eyepatch and did not put on the glasses. Suddenly, I saw only one of him! I almost jumped out of my seat screaming, 'I'm cured!' He started walking across the room, and I realised that I was not cured. In fact, I was worse than ever. His 'double' was about fifteen feet behind him! My heart sank. It was so disappointing, I could have cried. I turned it to humour, instead.

I whispered to Colin what happened, and we both started laughing. I started to go into one of my infamous fits of laughter, with tears running down my face.

'I thought I was cured, Colin! Mais, non! Deux garçon!'

'Stop, darling,' he pleaded, laughing.

'He is so hot,' I said referring to our sexy buyer. 'Two of him *is* better, anyway! What is better than one garçon? Deux garçon!' We could barely catch our breath laughing.

The rest of my day was much the same. I sat in the same chair, feeling crazy sensations in my head and various stages of pain in my eyes. I tried my best to concentrate on the people in the front of the room, whilst closing one eye and taking notes. I managed to stay awake, which was more than I could say for a few of our colleagues from France and Italy.

That night, we arrived back at our hotel around 7 p.m. We had dinner plans at 8 p.m. at a swanky restaurant called Café Marly. I had heard wonderful things about this restaurant from a Parisian guy I knew in London.

Alone in my room, I looked at the bed with longing. I had another argument with myself. *Sick Marlo* said, 'No way are you going out. You look like shit, and you will get in that bed!' *Fun Marlo* said, 'Why should everyone else have fun? It is not fair for you. You probably have a brain tumour. You could be dead in a few months! This could be your only chance to have fun in Paris.' That was the thought that got me to go.

Again, I truly don't know how I pulled myself together, but I did. I put on loads of makeup, a tight dress, heels, and the *Zorro* patch. My colleagues thought my look was very sexy, so I went with it.

The restaurant was superb: red walls, candles, very chic! I promised myself that I would not drink, not that I drink much, anyway. I thought it might have a negative effect on my vision. That was probably the least of my problems. Everyone else was drinking, smoking, and laughing. How I wished I could be one of them that night. How I wished I were not on this weird ride in Wonderland.

When our meals came, and I picked up my fork, I realised something very scary. I had no sense of where my mouth was. I knew it was on my face, of course, yet I lacked the normal sense we all have of where to put your food. I would like to say it was the strangest feeling I ever felt, but sadly, the 'strange feeling list' is long and growing. It was bizarre, though. I felt extremely self-conscious.

Everyone was smiling and talking, and I was having this wacky internal conversation. I was telling myself *You can do it. Watch the fork, slowly.* At this point, the room and everyone in it became background noise. This was a showdown between my fork and me. I watched the fork as I picked up two pieces of penne pasta. I carefully inserted the prongs of the fork into each tube of pasta, hence maximising the pasta's chance of staying on the fork.

I tried to watch the fork as it got closer to my mouth, but that was difficult to do without crossing my eyes. I brought my left hand up to touch my mouth quickly, so that I could feel where it was without people noticing that I was doing something weird.

It was difficult to eat like that, and I quickly got fed up with it. I started to wish that I had stayed in the hotel room. At least there I could order room service. *Perhaps I could just put the plate on the floor and eat like a dog in peace. At this point, what difference does it make?*

I decided that I needed a drink pronto. I ordered champagne, the one drink that makes me intoxicated after two sips. *Fantastique!*

I don't smoke, but I decided that I needed a cigarette too. I drank the champagne, smoked cigarettes, and started to have a great time! I calmed down so much. I ate maybe four bites of food the entire night. That was all I could stand without risking flinging it onto someone's jacket. It didn't matter anymore, though. I was no longer hungry and I was quickly getting drunk.

For a few minutes I forgot my troubles and started to enjoy my life again. For a few minutes I was in Paris drinking, smoking, and laughing in a chic restaurant. I considered myself a lucky girl.

After dinner, everyone decided that instead of taking a taxi, we would walk back to the hotel and enjoy the Parisian sky. *Why not?* I thought. *I am past exhaustion now anyway.* The walk back to the hotel was surreal, because at night, I would see lights blend into one another. It was a bit psychedelic.

It was like walking through wet canvas. The lights were all smeary and dreamy around me. It was somehow OK because I was drunk this time. I could smell the nicotine and alcohol on my breath, accompanied by the sweet smell of Paris at night. We walked by the Louvre museum and I didn't even know it. I just put one leg in front of the other and went where I was guided to go. I had the assistance of my lovely colleagues. An arm to lean on is a blessing and

I had several. They walked me back to the hotel like the little old auntie I had become.

The trip concluded the next day with more gruelling meetings. I did not bother with my eye experiments that day. I was much too tired and tried to concentrate on not throwing up from exhaustion.

We all took the train back to London that evening. Everyone was tired. My head felt so weird. Something about the sound of train rides has always made me go into deep thought. In fact, I've written many songs on trains. My mind was now in very deep thought. I was thinking how I was not the person I used to be. I felt some part of me dying inside. *How did this weird feeling ever happen? Why did it happen?* I closed my eyes, wondering to myself if I was going to die soon. *Is something going to explode in my head? Will I die quickly or slowly? At least I got to see Paris, even if it was not with William.*

Utter Despair

The night I got home from Paris, I opened a letter from the National Neurological Hospital that said I was scheduled for an MRI. The only problem was that it was scheduled for the 26th of November and I was leaving for a holiday in New York on the 24th. I was so upset. I rang the hospital to reschedule. I thought perhaps by some miracle, there might be a cancellation, and there was! There was an opening two days later! I was very lucky! The woman on the phone was kind and understanding. As anyone who visits doctors a lot knows, things are less stressful if the receptionist is pleasant.

The day of the appointment came. I went alone because not only am I an *awkward bitch* but I am a stubborn bitch too. Doing things on my own was always important to me, and now that I had something wrong with me, it was somehow even more important. William insisted that he go with me, but I told him that he couldn't go to every single appointment with me. If he did, he would never go to work. I told him I would be happier, both financially and mentally, if he went to work instead.

The building where I had the MRI was in Queen Square. This is a lovely part of London. It is literally a pretty square with gardens, fenced in by iron gates. Beautiful Victorian buildings surround the square.

The outside of the building was old and quaint, but inside it was state of the art. I was immediately impressed, and I felt comfortable there. Even the waiting room had a professional sophistication that I associate with New York.

A technician called me in to a cubicle, where I had to answer various health questions. She explained to me what the MRI machine was like. She explained that it makes a series of loud mechanical-type noises while you are in it. I had an MRI once when I was a teenager, so I didn't feel nervous about being put in the enclosed tunnel once again. She left me alone in the room for a few minutes to get changed into a dressing gown.

During that time alone, I had a conversation with myself (unusual, I know). *You know that there is something wrong with you, and you must find out what it is. Knowing is better than not knowing. They will probably find lesions all over your brain, and you will deal with it. Oh my*

God! Lesions! There could be lesions growing as I sit here! OK, breathe. Get hold of yourself.

The technician came back in what seemed like a month, but I am sure it was two minutes. She brought me into a large sterile room. It was barren except for the gigantic machine in the middle of it. This was the machine that I would be slid into like a pizza in a brick oven.

Another technician put me on the gurney-type table, tucked me under a warm blanket, and slid me in. It was freezing cold inside! Even with the warm blanket, I started shaking from the first second. The technician spoke to me through speakers inside the machine. 'You are going to hear a series of loud noises,' she said. 'This is normal.'

Loud? For anyone who has ever been inside an MRI, you know that they are not joking when they say 'loud'. I didn't remember my other MRI being this loud, but I guess it was. It sounded like I was inside a tumble dryer, but instead of tumbling with clothes, I was tumbling with a couple of wrenches and some loose nuts and bolts.

I began to block the noise. I started thinking to myself, *OK, lesions, now you can't hide. Show yourselves, you little fuckers.* Then I flipped back to the thoughts of a tumour again and I started to feel sick. I decided to not think any of these thoughts and go down a different trail of thought.

I took a mental trip to Las Vegas. I could hear the technician's voice float in and out of the splashing sounds at the pool. The hot sun felt good. I was having a great time with my sister Lorraine. I was tan and healthy, wearing my favourite metallic Chanel bathing suit and drinking a Starbucks double shot out of a can. Lorraine and I were discussing what posh restaurant we would eat at that night. This was a scene from an actual holiday. I was reliving it in vivid detail. How fabulous it was!

Then I heard, 'OK, Mrs. Parmelee, we're finished.'

What? What about Las Vegas? We haven't had dinner yet! We haven't even hit one slot machine! Oh no! I am not in Las Vegas. I am freezing on a cold slab, having a machine take pictures of my deteriorated brain. Yes, reality came flying back.

Anyone who has ever had any kind of test like this looks at the technician's face to see if he or she knows anything. It is human nature to try to probe into his or her mind. When the technician got me from the table, she started walking me to the door like I was her granny. She was extra gentle, holding on to my arms. I thought she was acting overly sympathetic. I was also paranoid. I wanted to beg her, 'Tell me! Tell me what you saw! Are there lesions? How many? Is there a tumour? Oh my God, is it the size of a grapefruit? Tell me, damn it! I know you know!'

Well, she told me nothing, of course. Now I was about to start the worst phase of all this: the waiting phase.

From there, I went straight to work and I tried to do things as normally as possible. People seemed to be acting nervous around me. I was trying to make people laugh, so that they would not feel sorry for me. Sympathy was the last thing I wanted. Everyone was concerned: William, my family, friends, co-workers. I think everyone thought that the worst was possible.

It was difficult that entire week. It was getting harder and harder to go up and down stairs. My four-inch heels were in my work locker for a while. Those heels were part of my Supergirl uniform. I could no longer be Supergirl, and that was not acceptable to me. I wanted to be the person I had been just months before.

So, in my usual stubborn fashion, I neglected breaks and put on the heels for the next few days. No matter how shitty I felt, I decided to push myself to the outer limits. I would not give in to whatever was wrong with me.

'What are you doing, Madam?' Colin asked, looking down at my feet.

'These heels are not as high as they look,' I said. 'They're platforms. I'll be fine.'

'This is coming from the woman who asked me yesterday if the walls had been painted pink,' he said. 'Oh yes, and the A4 paper turned pink as well.'

He was referring to a change in my vision that suddenly made all white things look pale pink. It was just another symptom to add to the list.

'Oh dear,' I said, giggling. 'I guess you're right. I'm not changing my shoes, though. What if Tom Ford comes in? I'm no Frumpa-doodle.'

Colin laughed as I said one of his favourite *Marlo* words. 'You're mad, woman.'

I clearly did push myself to the limit, because that weekend my eye problems began to worsen. The pain and the double vision got even worse. In the previous weeks, I had had one small field of vision that was normal, on the left side. If I looked at something on the extreme left and slightly down, I could see it normally. That was what I called my 'little window'. I would try to look through that little window as much as possible. Of course, doing this in public makes you look like you have some kind of physical problem that has left you cocking your head to one side.

Well, on Sunday, the 21st of November, my little window closed. That field of vision was now doubled as well. This really sucked, for lack of a better word. I felt like a cruel joke was being played on me. I was not sure how much more I could mentally take. I tried to hold my sanity together, but in private, I started snapping. I thought I was perhaps going insane.

At one point that Sunday, I tried to enjoy the weird feelings and the now worsened double vision. I thought, *People do pay good money to feel like this. I am going to enjoy it.* I started staring at my two selves in the mirror and singing songs.

'Look William, we are singing a duet!'

William laughed at first, but I think he was scared. I began referring to myself as *we*. There were physically two of me when I looked in the mirror, so why not? I had a new friend: *Marlo #2*. She was a nice girl. She looked just like me. We would do lots of dances together in the mirror. She was completely in sync with me. It was like synchronized swimming without the water or the pretty silver swim caps. We could also make our mouths move at the same time. My favourite time with her was when we did the 'YMCA' song.

William did not enjoy watching that one, though. He yelled at me. 'Enough!'

I guess he did not share my humour at the time, but if I did not laugh as much as I did, I would have cried. I guess, in a way, I was cracking up. William said that I had better stop the dancing and ring Moorfields instead. So that is what I did.

That Tuesday, I went back to see the neuro-ophthalmologist at Moorfields Eye Hospital.

William wanted to come with me to the appointment, but again, I insisted that I go alone. We were leaving for New York the next day and I did not want him to miss any more work because of my stupid problems.

I was sitting in the waiting room for about a half-hour, listening to other people's conversations as usual. But this day was a turning point for me. I was about to hear something that would change my life.

In the waiting room, there was a young woman who was about my age. She was sitting with her mother, who looked to be about seventy years of age. There was a walking stick in between them. I assumed the stick was her mother's, even though I learned early on in the conversation that the daughter was the patient.

A woman sitting across from them was asking them which doctor they were seeing and how long they had gone to him. These were all boring questions, until she asked the woman what symptoms she had. The mother spoke on the daughter's behalf. She began telling a story that was all too familiar.

'She suddenly woke up one day with a little blurry vision. It came out of nowhere. Then it went into double vision,' she said. 'Her toes went numb as well.'

I couldn't believe my ears! She was telling *my* story! I almost felt elated. I could not believe that someone had such a similar set of problems to me. This was great news. I thought, *I have what she has!*

The doctor came out and called the young woman's name. She reached for the walking stick and struggled to get out of her chair. She inched along at the speed of a turtle. She put one foot a couple of inches in front of the other. Her hand was shaking as she gripped the stick. Her head was slightly cocked to the side. This was a familiar stance, as she must have been struggling to look through *her* small window of vision.

It took her ages to get to the examining area. My heart sank to my stomach watching her. I was still getting over the fact that the stick belonged to her and not her mother. Seeing her struggle like that hit me hard. She was too young to have to go through this. I started to wonder what her life was like. It must have been difficult.

My attention was taken off her when I heard the other woman ask the girl's mother another question. 'What does your daughter have?'

'Multiple sclerosis,' her mother answered.

Her words rang in my ears like the bells of Notre Dame. My world crashed. Everything fell to shit for me. My blood pressure soared. My breathing became shallow. I started to have a full-blown panic attack in the waiting room. My legs felt like tree stumps. I became frozen with fear and panic. My thoughts became fast and erratic. *I have multiple sclerosis, and I will not be able to walk soon. I will not be able to see, either. I will slowly become a vegetable. I have MS.*

There was no way I didn't have it. There was no one who could convince me otherwise.

When the doctor finally called my name, I did not think I could move out of the seat. I was rigid. I don't know how I got up. I went into autopilot at that point. I wanted to start screaming as I walked into the examination room. After the panic attack, I was not sure how I could sit still while he looked at me.

He examined me to make sure that there was no bleeding behind my eyes. There was not. He told me to just continue wearing the glasses and it would eventually resolve itself. There were no results back from any of the blood tests or MRI yet, so there was nothing more to do. There was an unspoken feeling in the office. Maybe he knew that it was likely to be MS, maybe he didn't. I did not ask what he thought. I did not want to know what he thought. I left the office holding back tears. I was in a daze.

I was due in work after my appointment. I tried not to cry on the tube ride there. When I got near work, I wandered into a Starbucks to comfort myself with my beloved Caramel Macchiato. As I sat there, I told myself, *You are Marlo. You are still the same person, but now you have multiple sclerosis.*

Looking around at other people, I imagined what it would be like to be them. I wanted to be someone else: maybe the man next to me, sipping his latté and reading a book. I wondered if he had any ailments. I looked over at a woman sitting by the door reading over notes, probably from a meeting. *I could be her. She doesn't look like she has any diseases. Unlike me.*

I let an hour go by and then I got up and walked to work. When my colleagues asked how the appointment went, I burst out crying. I was a shambles. I told them about the woman in the waiting room and how I knew that I had the same disease. They kept assuring me that I did not. They were very comforting, but in my heart, I knew the truth.

Every part of me knew it. The fact seemed to be that if it wasn't MS, then it was something worse. People try their best to comfort you, but sometimes you just know what you know. Instinct tells us a lot, and you should always trust it.

I continued my day, feeling disconnected from life. With every task, I felt some part of me slipping away. I felt the *old Marlo* was about to die, and I was planning her funeral. I felt so alone and in utter despair.

New York to Miami

The day after that, William and I flew to New York for our Thanksgiving holiday. I was glad to be going home. A tiny part of me was still thinking that a tumour was a possibility. If that were the case, then I wanted to die in the house I grew up in, the house where my father died.

On the plane, I had the fear that my brain might bleed from the pressure of the altitude. I was thinking so many ridiculous thoughts. Your mind can play many tricks on you when your future is uncertain.

Our families were overjoyed to see William and me. This was a stressful time for them. It was not easy for them to be living so far away from us. They had to hear over the phone about every symptom and the results of every appointment I had. I know they were anxious to see if I looked sick. They all liked the granny glasses, actually. Some people were upset when I put the eyepatch on, and some thought it looked cool. I guess it freaked some of them out. It was too extreme. Glasses are more acceptable. My mom could see that I did not look as well as usual, but other people were fooled by the red lip gloss and bronzing powder.

Many people said, 'You don't look sick.'

Well, I was not going to visit people I had not seen in months and allow myself to look like shit. People assume that if you don't look shitty, then you are not sick. I guess this is human nature too.

Usually on and around Thanksgiving, I go into tirades about the white man's pillage and destruction of the indigenous American people. 'Happy kill the American Indian Day,' I used to say. 'We are not the real Americans! Red men are the only true Americans.' Every year I go on about the same thing, but this time I was not feeling energetic enough to give my speech.

My health was now the main topic of conversation. Everyone had some sort of opinion about my problems. Some thought that my ailments had to be stress related. Others thought it was a virus. It certainly could not be anything serious. I told a few people that I thought it was MS, but they did not agree. They told me that I was thinking the worst and letting my imagination run away with me. I was too young and healthy. Even my mother-in-law, who is a nurse, said I did not have MS. That was the *mom* speaking and not the nurse, though.

There was another issue brewing also. My immediate family felt that the medical attention I was receiving in England was too slow. I assured them that things went as quickly as possible. My sister Lisa suggested that I ring someone at Moorfields and ask them to fax the results of the MRI and blood tests. This way, I would not have to wait more weeks to find out what the tests revealed.

In a way, I did not want to know the results. I wanted to be on a holiday away from myself, but I rang anyway. I was referred to a secretary of the Mister, who said she could fax the results when they came in. We waited several days and heard nothing. I rang again and left a message. This kind of chasing up results was common in England, and I was embarrassed that my family had to witness it. This added fuel to their argument that I was not receiving the best-possible care in England.

Another upsetting issue came up. I was sad that I could not drive a car on that holiday. I was accustomed to driving everywhere.

'What a joke this is,' I said to my mom. 'Me! The one who used to drive everywhere and anywhere! New York City at two in the morning! Florida to New Orleans in middle of the night! Now, I have to rely on rides from other people just to go to the grocery store!'

My mom tried to console me. 'You'll drive again when your eyes get better. You've driven people around for years. Let them drive you now.'

William kept saying, 'I'll take you anywhere you want to go.' He wanted to take me shopping or to friends' houses, but I felt guilty. I wanted him to enjoy his holiday, not chauffeur me around. I felt so damn tired anyway. I really did not want to go anywhere until my sister Lorraine came up with a plan.

She suggested that we take a jaunt to Miami for sun and fun. This idea made something spark in me. I thought it was a great idea. If we went, I would be able to relax and catch up with her, and William could have a few days away from me. I felt like he needed it but just didn't know it. He was so supportive, but I knew he needed a break from all this drama.

Lorraine and I flew down to Miami and stayed at the Loews Hotel. It was fantastic. We had taken dozens of holidays together throughout the years. One thing we always do on our holidays is laugh hysterically for no reason at all. I mean we laugh out of control. We laugh until tears are rolling down our faces and we are gasping for air.

We made so many sick and inappropriate jokes about my crisis. While waiting for food service on the beach, I would say things like, 'Can you please hurry, my tumour is growing, and time is of the essence.' We had such a giggle.

I told Lorraine, 'I have done four major cities (London, New York, Paris, and Miami) in a span of one week, and I'm half blind and disoriented! How many people can say that?'

'You're right,' she said. 'Not many people. You are doing very well!'

I was proud of myself. I thoroughly relaxed on the beach. It was not too hot, and there was a cool breeze. It was superb.

The first night in Miami we went to a trendy restaurant on Ocean Drive. They served amazing cocktails with neon glowing ice cubes. These drinks looked even more psychedelic when I took my glasses off! I was terribly embarrassed by the glasses that night. Here were all these trendy South Beach people, and there was I, the usually fabulous Marlo, now reduced to granny glasses and a blind eye. My sister insisted that I looked like a trendsetter who happened to be wearing glasses. I guess she was right, because we got invited to a private party on the rooftop.

'Are you up to going?' Lorraine asked.

'Yes, why not?' I joked. 'I am drunk and blind, and hey, there's a pool. Sounds like a recipe for disastrous fun!'

We went up to the party, and the pool was actually more of a navigational nightmare than anticipated, so we had to leave.

On the way back to the hotel, a couple stopped to ask me directions to a different hotel. Lorraine let out a small laugh, as she knows about my invisible 'Need directions? Ask me!' sign on my forehead. She saved me, and gave the directions, as it was a hotel we had just walked by.

'Isn't it crazy?' I asked Lorraine, who was still laughing. 'No matter what freakin' city....'

On our second day in Miami, something extraordinary happened. I woke up with normal vision! I called over to Lorraine in her bed.

'Are you awake, Lorraine? I have some great news! I can see!'

It was like something out of a film. 'It's a miracle! I can see! I can see!'

She got excited, because she thought I was cured. I did, too, come to think of it. I was certain that the sun gods had bestowed some South Beach Miracle upon me. Room service was on its way and I was looking forward to seeing my food clearly!

Sadly, the clear vision only lasted for about twenty minutes, so by the time the food arrived, the double vision was back. We were disappointed, but we did not let that stop the fun. Besides, instead of twenty-four-hour shit vision, I now had only twenty-three hours and forty minutes of shit vision. Lorraine said that this was 'a definite improvement' and that it was a sign that things were getting better.

'You're right,' I said. 'I will focus on the positive.'

I shrugged off the initial disappointment. The positive of that day was that I had another designer bathing suit to show off and yet another pair of sandals. We enjoyed our usual day of laughter and people-watching at the beach. From the looks of things in South Beach, I was not the only disoriented girl in head-to-toe Chanel. There were some interesting characters.

At Emeril's restaurant that night, the waiter was seating me on the left side of Lorraine, meaning I would have to look to my right to see her. This was something I could not do. I told him I had to sit on the other side of her. He looked at me like I was being difficult.

'I'm blind in the right eye,' I quickly lied.

'Oh! Are you really? Sorry,' he said, and then happily accommodated me.

I was learning that little white lies came in handy. Besides, it is too hard to explain to someone my exact ailments. Saying, 'blind in one eye' or 'partially blind in one eye' is much easier.

When I woke the next morning, I could see normally once again! Room service had just brought us breakfast, and I was able to see two eggs instead of four. The joy of looking down at my meal and seeing it properly made me want to scream with happiness! I can't accurately describe how good it felt to sit on our terrace; eating breakfast and watching the ships come in. I could actually see the ships clearly! In fact, I had no idea that Lorraine had been watching the ships the two previous mornings. I did not know they were there.

That morning, I felt like I had won a game show. The good vision lasted for about forty minutes this time. After that, it slowly started to go back to double.

'It's all falling to shit again, Lorraine.'

We were disappointed all over again, but I had gained twenty more minutes of my life. Lorraine tried to cheer me up.

'Don't worry,' she assured me. 'You gained more time. You *are* improving!'

I told Lorraine that I was pretty certain that I had MS, and she actually agreed with me! She was the first person to do so. She had been reading up on it extensively, as had my whole family. Lisa thought that it was *probably* MS, but did not want to say anything for sure until we got the MRI results back. My sister Colleen and my mom thought anything was possible but hoped for the best.

Lorraine agreed that I seemed to have the symptoms. I had so many symptoms that I would have never linked together. That is one of the difficulties with this disease. There are so many signs that seem unrelated at first. It is easy to go to the doctor and not mention half of them. I had pins and needles so many times and just assumed that I slept wrong. It felt comforting to have someone agree with me and still think I would be OK.

Flying to Miami was a good idea. Spending time with Lorraine was therapeutic. The entire break was sublime. By the end of it, I had gained an hour of clear vision a day. That was certainly progress, and it made me very happy. We figured that by now the results of my MRI would be in, and we headed back to New York.

The results had not been faxed. When I listened to my messages on my answerphone in London, I realised that another secretary had rung to say that I needed to sign a consent form for the fax. I quickly wrote out a consent letter and faxed it to her. Days passed and she still did not fax the results. In the end, the holiday was over, and no fax had arrived.

It was now the 6th of December and I felt that not knowing for one more week was not going to kill me. My family members were a bit angry, I think. They wanted to know. They were having a tough time not knowing, and I think that they were secretly thinking the worst all the time. Somehow a few more days of not knowing seemed appealing to me. *Besides,* I thought, *if it was MS, they would contact me.* Here's a word to the wise: if the results lean towards MS, they don't always contact you.

D-Day

઼

The 13th of December was the day of my appointment with the neuro-ophthalmologist at Moorfields Eye Hospital. Because it was in the afternoon, I decided to go to work in the morning. This took my mind off of the appointment for a few minutes. My colleagues were a bit nervous. So was I. As I left work, everyone wished me good luck.

'I know they are going to say that I have MS. I know it,' I told them.

'Think positive,' everyone said.

I am thinking positive, I thought.

On the tube ride to the hospital, I started pondering the thought of not going. Once again, I wished I was someone else, on my way to somewhere else. The thought of a tumour returned, but then I thought, *Wouldn't they have called immediately? No,* I thought, *it is not a tumour. It is MS. I definitely have MS.*

Another thought occurred to me. *What if they say that they don't know what is wrong? This would actually be worse than MS. At least with a diagnosis, I can face it. I can't fight an enemy who is invisible. If I know what it is, I can fight it.*

I arrived at the clinic and met William and my cousin, Kerry, who wanted to be there for added support. When the doctor called me, I thought, *This is it.*

The three of us trailed behind him single file like prisoners walking into a courtroom to receive our sentencing.

He began by examining me the same way he had in all the other visits. He started asking me about my symptoms. He wanted to know if I felt any better, if my vision had improved, and so on. I thought about screaming, 'Do I have MS or not? I can't wait another minute!' Then I thought, *Well, if I had MS, he would have said it already.*

He then asked me if anyone had phoned me with the MRI results yet. I knew that was not a good question, and then the tumour thought reared its head again. My face started to heat up.

'No one rang,' I answered slowly.

He took out the results from my MRI scan, and said, 'You have multiple lesions on your brain that are typical of multiple sclerosis.'

The sense of relief that came over me was incredible. No one wants to hear that they have an incurable disease of the brain and nervous system, but I felt relief just the same.

I heard William exhale. Kerry did the same. I looked at their faces. William's eyes were filled with tears. I could see his mouth shaking slightly, trying to hold back more tears. Kerry looked like she was in shock; her cheeks were flushed and her eyes were tearing. They both wanted to console me, but I think at that moment, it was *I* who needed to console *them.*

The doctor explained to me that I would no longer be attending the eye hospital. Instead, I would be going to the National Hospital for Neurology and Neurosurgery.

'So this means I graduated?' I joked.

'Cum laude,' he said. By this time, three other doctors had come over who were all looking at me. One looked like he was fresh out of medical school. One was the Mister. He was a wise Mister, because I believe he suspected all along that I had MS. The other doctor standing there was the young one who thought I had migraines. I felt like saying, 'Some migraine, huh?'

I left the clinic with two feelings: relief for knowing what I had, and an underlying grief because things would never be the same. I was in better shape than my husband and cousin, though. They walked out with heavy hearts.

They kept telling me how brave I was. This was not bravery. This was just life.

The first thing I wanted to do was ring my mom, which I did from my mobile phone. I had to tell her straight away. I know she was nervous to hear how the appointment went. She had been praying so much for me. In fact, all her friends were praying for me. My sisters were praying. My aunties, uncles, cousins, and friends were praying (in America, Ireland, and England). They were all waiting to hear the news from my mom. I thought, *God, this is going to be the diagnosis 'heard round the world'. My poor mom.*

I wanted to offer her immediate consolation from her disappointment. I wanted her to hear that my voice was strong and so was my spirit. I wanted her to know that all the prayers *did* work. I was fine and I would always be fine.

I broke the news to Colleen, who answered the phone. I could hear her heart sink into her stomach. My mom got on the line for a three-way conversation. She sounded stronger, though she was very upset.

'Are the doctors certain?' they both asked. It was a harder blow for them to hear this over the phone. Living far away always makes things worse.

'We're coming over, right Mom?' Colleen said. 'We'll be there for you. What do you need us to bring?'

'Yes, we'll get our plane ticket when we hang up with you,' my mom said.

'No,' I commanded. 'It is not necessary and I don't want you coming all the way over here for this. It's done.'

I felt that whatever was going to happen was now set in stone. There was nothing anyone could do.

So, you've just been told that you have an incurable disease (or a *condition,* as it's called in the UK) and you've broken the news to your family. What do you do next? You have a bloody drink. We headed over to a pub. Gin and tonic might be the cure for MS, for all we know.

'Should you be drinking?' William asked.

'At this point, does it matter?' I answered.

After only one round, we started getting silly.

'I have lesions,' I said and started laughing. 'I have lesions on my brain. Better yet, I have *pictures* of the lesions on my brain as well! Jesus Christ.'

'We should name them,' Kerry suggested. It might sound absurd—well it is absurd—but it sounded like a great idea at the time.

'Let's call one *Abigail,*' she suggested. She chose this name for no particular reason. The whole idea made her and me roar with laughter.

'Abigail? I fucking love it,' I said as if I was hearing the most brilliant idea ever.

William did not share our disturbed sense of humour.

'You guys are nuts,' he said, but he was laughing a little too. Kerry and I were falling off our chairs laughing. From that moment on, my lesions were sometimes referred to as 'Abigail and her friends'.

I felt elated. I felt the need to tell everyone I ever met. 'Hey! I've been feeling crazy for months and it's not because I am insane! I have a disease that causes people to feel this way! I am not alone! I am one of many!'

I wanted to do something drastic. Who knows what? I felt like there was a reason I got this stupid disease, and I was going to find that reason. I was not going to let this stop me from living my life the way I wanted to live it. I was not going to let this stop me from being my glamorous, red-lipped, musica-fashionista self. Slamming my glass down after another swig, I declared, 'I am not letting this stop me. I am going to leave my mark on this city if it fucking kills me!'

We all raised our glasses. 'Hallelujah! Amen.'

Jubilation

&

The gin and tonic wore off the next day, but oddly enough, the feelings of relief and jubilation did not. I was somehow satisfied that I was correct in my own diagnosis. The diagnosis validated my feelings and symptoms. In the prior months, I had felt like I was losing my mind more than a few times. Now I had a solid medical reason for my feelings.

'Are you all right?' William asked that morning, snuggling me close.

'I am great!' I said.

'I will always take care of you,' he said. 'You know that, don't you?'

'I know,' I answered.

I marched into work ready to tell everyone about my diagnosis. By the pensive looks on their faces, I could tell that some of my colleagues were afraid to ask me how the doctor's visit went. They greeted me with nervous hellos and then started chatting about the new jackets that had arrived, the nasty boots a client was wearing, and the weather: everything that wasn't the dreaded doctor's visit.

Now I felt like I was about to disappoint them, and that made me feel guilty. In my mind, I was somehow letting people down. Here they were, telling me the day before that they knew I'd bring good news. Yet here I am today telling them crap news.

The first person I told was Simon. His response was quick. He said, 'Don't worry, my brother has it, and he's fine. You'll be fine too.' He flashed a little smile. He looked down, shuffled his papers around, and then looked back to me as if to say, 'Right, let's look at our targets for the day, shall we?' He acted a little nonchalant about the whole thing.

I was taken aback by his reaction. I did not want people to burst into sympathetic tears, but I also thought that the matter required a bit more tenderness than that. I would later find out that Simon did not have much communication with that particular brother, which aided in his lack of understanding of MS.

The UK area manager, Simon's boss, came into the store that morning. He was the man who had originally hired me and was quite fond of me. He was visibly upset by my news. His eyes started to well up with tears when I told him.

'Are they 100 per cent positive? Do you think they might have misdiagnosed you?' he asked.

'No, I don't think they misdiagnosed me,' I said.

'Are you OK? Are you *sure* you're OK?

'I'm perfectly fine.' I kept answering.

'You're very brave,' he said.

'Believe me, I am not brave,' I said. 'Fire-fighters are brave; people who have choices are brave. I don't have a choice, do I? I can't pretend I don't have it. I have to get on with things.'

I could see his face was still saddened, so I tried to make him laugh, saying, 'I am not going to stay home and whine, especially when there are new clothes to buy!'

That morning, I proceeded to tell the rest of the staff. Colin, not surprisingly, was the most supportive. He hugged me and told me he was there if I needed anything. Everyone reacted in different ways, but each one was supportive. For various reasons, many people did not understand what it was.

One reason was language. Because English was not the first language of many people at work, I had to learn how to say multiple sclerosis in several languages. 'I have *sclérose en plaques.' Oh mon Dieu!*

I would later find out that many people who have MS (or MSers, as we are called) do not tell their employers they have it. For me, withholding this information would have been damn near impossible. Because I had turned into the awkward bitch right before their eyes, I would not have been comfortable trying to hide the fact that I had MS. Plus, if I dare say, I do have a big mouth, so keeping this a secret would have been doubly hard for me.

I subconsciously 'decided' that I would never be in a wheelchair, but I knew that I would probably be unwell at other times in the future. If my co-workers saw me wobbling around and clinging onto railings, they would start to think the wrong thing, like I was drunk or drugged, as some had thought previously. I preferred that people just knew the truth. It was less mentally tiring for me that way.

Plus, I needed to vent to people at certain times. The formidable TV host Anne Robinson came in on a day when I could not see well. She asked me to pin her trousers! I was in a sweat looking for someone to help me, as the tailor had the day off. There was no one available, and there was Anne, waiting by the mirror. I had no choice. *You can do this*, I convinced myself, as I got down on my knees.

I don't think she noticed that my head was very close to the ground, as I closed one eye and put my face next to the hem of her trousers! I did it though, and I did it well. When Anne left (she was very nice, by the way) I immediately ran to Colin to show him my pinning.

'Well done,' he said. 'Better than I would've done, darling.'

'Yes,' I agreed. 'One point for the disability team!'

I began emailing all my friends in the States to tell them my news that I had MS. The reactions were all different. Some were supportive. Some were shocked. Others were blasé. Laura, of course, was one of the supportive ones. I know she was sad for me, but she felt that I would be OK. She started to clip newspaper articles about therapies for MS. She told her parents about my diagnosis, and they bought me a book that helped their friend who also had MS. Those reactions made me feel comforted.

Others were not so comforting. One wrote back, 'Oh no! Whatever you do don't get pregnant! My cousin has MS and had a baby. She then got worse than ever!'

'Gee,' I wrote back. 'Thanks for that terrific advice.'

I received an apology email from him. He laughed out loud (LOL) from embarrassment and wrote that he was sorry for his outburst.

Although reactions were all different, one thing my friends had in common was that they either didn't know exactly what MS was or they had the wrong idea about it. Everyone had heard of it, but pretty much all of them asked me to tell them exactly what it was.

I realised that I did not have all the answers I thought I had either. Lisa had given me a lot of information about MS, and to add to that, she bought several books, read them from cover to cover, and then sent them to me with the highlights she had made! She practises Eastern medicine as well as Western, so her book selection included alternative therapy books.

Reading those books was just the beginning. I began to immerse myself in dedicated research. I was like a student preparing for an MS-related dissertation. I spent countless hours on every MS-related site known to man. Some were reputable and had great information. Others were completely misinformed nonsense and I was sorry that I stumbled onto them. It was all trial and error.

After looking at dozens upon dozens of sites, it became easier to distinguish the reputable ones from the others. The MS Society's websites were very useful. They had an area for newly diagnosed people. This was very handy and also made me feel like I was one of many people who had this disease.

I started signing up onto MS chatrooms and websites. I found a great website called Jooly's Joint, which I immediately became a member of. I was proactive and bursting with positive energy about beating this disease.

I started to understand exactly what the disease does and how it can progress. I understood what myelin was and how the immune system accidentally attacks it. Our nerves are like a system of wires throughout the body. They are made up of nerve cells that are connected by fibres called axons. Axons send nerve impulses, telling the body to pick up a glass, for example. Myelin is the layer of fatty lipids and proteins that protects these axons like insulation.

In MS, the immune system attacks the myelin, causing this insulation to become inflamed. That inflammation can either heal or leave scars. Multiple sclerosis actually means 'multiple scars'. When these scars occur, there is a break in the nerve impulses. For example, the message of picking up a glass gets slowed down or faulted. What happens? You break half your glass set, like me. Two highballs, two wine glasses, four small glasses, five champagne glasses (yes, five!), and three cups, all smashed accidentally. But who's counting?

I read about why people with MS have it so differently. It all seems to depend on what nerve or nerves are damaged by the lesions. Not everyone with MS has lesions in the same area. In fact, no two people have it the same. I was able to visualise where my lesions were, and I made the connection between where the lesions were and where my problems were.

I also understood that there were different types of MS and that they each had names. The type I had was called *relapsing-remitting multiple sclerosis*. This basically means that there are periods of relapse, where symptoms flare up, and there are periods of remission, when the symptoms either go away or get a lot better. Apparently, as time goes on, the chances are that the damage progresses and the nerves no longer heal as quickly or completely. When there are less obvious relapses and recoveries, the disease goes into another stage, where the damage is progressive. That frightened the hell out of me.

One website suggested that newly diagnosed people should not worry about ending up in a wheelchair, because 'only' one out of five people with MS ever needs to use a wheelchair at some stage. *Well*, I thought, *if one out of five people won the lottery, millions more would play!* Is one out of five a comforting ratio? Not in my book.

The more I read about MS, the more I saw it as a foe that I needed to learn how to fight. I already knew that there was no cure yet for MS. Those two words together—'no' and 'cure'—had stood out in the weeks prior when I suspected that I could have MS.

I have felt that time was against me since I was a child. I have always felt that my life was working against the deadline of death. Throughout my life, I had put a lot of pressure on myself to write songs, visit places, experience life, all before it was too late. Now that I had MS, that feeling was doubled. I now had something inside me that could potentially slow me down, or even worse, stop me in my tracks. Time was truly not on my side.

My ray of hope was that there were four drugs out on the market that could slow this disease down. Yes, there was no cure so far, but these drugs, called beta interferons and Copaxone, all taken by injection, could potentially slow it down by up to 30 per cent. They were being used for the type of multiple sclerosis I had: relapsing-remitting.

For me, even slowing it down 5 per cent was worth it, and I was keen to start taking one of these drugs straight away. The fact that it was an injection didn't really bother me. I would have eaten cow dung if someone said that it slowed MS down by 30 per cent.

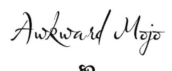

Awkward Mojo

&

When you learn that you have MS, you start hearing of other people who have it. I have found that many people either know someone or know a person who knows another person who has it.

It was now Christmas time. Colin wrote me a Christmas card that read, 'Have a prism-tastic Christmas!'

'How dare you mock my eye problems! I have a disability,' I said, laughing. I thought it was a wonderful card (I still have it as a keepsake.)

He got serious then and said, 'My mum has a good friend with MS.'

'Really?' I asked.

'Yes. I was telling my mum about your diagnosis and she rang her friend straight away. Her name is Carol. She told my mum she would like to talk to you.'

'She would?' I asked, completely scared and intrigued.

'You would like her,' he said. 'She's a bit like you. She's feisty. She always makes us laugh. My mum used to work with her.' He paused while he thought for a moment. 'I forgot to get Carol's number from my mum, but you know what, Marlo? I am going to ring her now and get the number.'

Within minutes of learning about this woman Carol, I had her phone number in my hand. All I knew was that she was a quick-witted individual and that she also had MS. I felt comfort sweep over me.

I decided to ring Carol that weekend. Even though she was expecting my phone call, I was a bit nervous to ring her. I picked up the phone several times and hung up before completely dialling her number. I practised what I would say:

'Hi Carol, we've never met, but I heard your brain has lesions too!'

Or maybe I would say, 'Hi Carol, I am Marlo. I heard you would like to speak with me considering the fact that I have what you have.'

I finally managed to pull myself together and dial the number. Her husband answered the phone. I worried that he was probably wondering what this person with an American accent wanted with his wife. I feared that he thought I was a cold caller claiming they won a trip to Florida. He paused for a moment and then told me Carol was not well and could not come to the phone.

I felt like I had interrupted something. I was so embarrassed. I told him my name and that I had MS as well. That was why Colin's mom had given me her name and number. I could hear that he understood, as his tone changed. Suddenly, saying that I had MS was like a secret password to getting through. He told me she would ring me back when she felt better, so I left him my number.

Carol, or *Carol the fabulous*, as I now think of her, rang back a few hours later. She told me she was sick, but not from MS. She had the flu. She wanted to talk to me because, well, she had a lot to say.

Carol inspired me. She is a clever woman and is not afraid to tell it to you like it is. She is witty and filled with fire. I got such a kick out of her. She told me not to be scared. She gave me advice on everything. Some of her best advice was about keeping a positive attitude.

'If you keep a positive attitude, you will not get sicker,' she said. 'Tell yourself what I told myself: I will never be in a wheelchair.'

I agreed with everything Carol said. She was stubborn as a mule. She was probably more stubborn than I was. I enjoyed our conversation so much. She told me that she was going to get me information on alternative treatments that she had received at an 'MS centre' near her. She explained that there were several of these centres throughout the UK. They were charity-run centres where people with MS could receive alternative therapies. She said she couldn't remember where she put the phone number, joking that it was because the MS made her forget things.

'Blame it *all* on MS,' she said laughing. 'That's what I do.'

Our conversation lasted for at least an hour, if not more. We started our chat as complete strangers with one thing in common, and we ended it as friends. She said she would ring me when she found the phone number.

Around the time I met Carol, I met another wonderful woman, called Magdalara. She and her partner Bruce, who is equally lovely, were clients of Yves Saint Laurent, and they had come in to the store a few times since I had been there. I had an immediate connection with them. They both dressed mostly in black. Magdalara was, and is, a beautiful woman with fair, luminous skin, blue eyes, and lips that were always painted some shade of ruby. Her hair was white-blonde and always in some modern short hairstyle. She looked impeccable.

Bruce had sleek, long, salt-and-pepper hair that was always pulled back into a neat ponytail. They reminded me of what William and I could grow up to look like, but there was something more than that. There was something mystical about them, and since our very first conversation, we felt like we were friends. Whenever I thought of Magdalara, she and Bruce would come in. In turn, whenever she thought of me, I would ring her. It was uncanny.

That week they came into the shop and we started having our usual fun chat.

'Are you OK?' Magdalara asked me.

'Yes, I'm very well,' I lied. 'How are you?'

Her reaction was that of someone who knows things. She said, 'I mean, are you *OK?*'

It was at that moment that I realised something that I had previously suspected. In fact, it was something Colin and I had discussed several times. I realised that she was psychic, or some type of spiritual mystic. (She is actually an incredibly gifted energy field consultant. *Google* it!)

Even though I was telling everyone of my diagnosis, I was not yet in the practice of telling clients, but she was different.

'I just found out that I have multiple sclerosis,' I admitted.

She nodded. 'I see,' she said, as if knowing that she was right about something.

We chatted some more about MS, shoes, fashion, and gardens. Before she left she came over to me and hugged me tightly. We had never even shaken hands before! She held my arms and looked me in the eyes. 'Because of what I do I can tell you that you are going to be fine,' she said. 'You *will* be fine.'

My hairs stood up on the back of my neck! 'Yes,' I whispered, 'I will be fine,' as I watched her smile at me and walk out of the shop. She infused a light of happiness into me that was indescribable.

My happiness continued for a few weeks. I even found a guitarist in that time! After all the terrible auditions months before, I decided it was time to give it another go, and I found a great guy very quickly. We had a couple of rehearsals and they went very well. Things were looking up!

The best part of it all was that my vision was slowly, but surely, returning to normal. I had several more appointments with Despina, the wonderful technician at Moorfields Eye Hospital, during this time. At each appointment, I was given a weaker prism, as my eyes got stronger. My frequent trips to Moorfields had become an unlikely comfort to me. I was getting better. Every time I went I followed the same routine of having the jacket potato after my visit. I would sit there in the cafeteria by myself and think of how lucky I was to be taken care of at such a good hospital. *These people really know their eyeballs.... and brains.*

I finally got to the point where I could see clearly without the glasses. There was just a small area to the right gaze which was a little doubled. This was a marked improvement, though. Even the weird feelings in my head were lessening. I wrote in my journal that I felt 'normal' for the first time in months! I had forgotten what it felt like to just feel like me. It was like I returned to my own body. I was back, and my fabulousness would soon be back in full force!

The real sign that my mojo was back was that construction workers were once again watching me walk by. There were many buildings getting worked on near my shop. Sadly, the construction workers had stopped looking at me in the prior weeks, a clear indication that my mojo was out of order. Now, I had it 'going on' once again!

As I walked by one of the sites, an older construction worker looked me up and down and said, 'Hello, love.'

'Good morning,' I answered. After all, one should be polite when spoken to.

This got the attention of some of the younger ones too, who started to say hello and smile. I smiled but pretended to be much too shy to look directly at them, as I started to walk a little less rushed and a little sexier. I wanted to enjoy my brief moment of feeling good about myself. As I walked down this *catwalk*, I noticed that one of the last audience members was particularly fit. I had to look that one directly in the eyes! He smiled at me and I felt unstoppable!

This wonderful feeling came just in time, because we had booked another Mantis and the Prayer gig for that month. This one was at a club called Embargo in Chelsea. William and I had invited a lot of people to this one, so we were excited. I felt a little anxious, though, because this was my first gig with the *knowledge* that I had MS.

For probably the first time in my life, I doubted my capabilities. I began wondering if I would lose feeling in my hands while I was playing. I thought maybe I would have a memory problem on stage and not know what to play. I kept thinking, *Am I going to fuck up this entire show? Oh my God, I might fall off the bloody stage.*

During the rehearsal earlier in the week, I noticed that although I was feeling great, a few minor things were wrong. If I were a robot, I would have said I was operating smoothly except for a few minor glitches.

There is a dial on my keyboard that I have to turn in the middle of a song to change the sound I use. Before MS, I used to be able to turn it fast and continue playing. In fact, I would keep playing with my left hand while I turned the knob with my right. Suddenly, this knob was my new nemesis. I could not make my hand steady enough to turn it with finesse. Unfortunately, if you turn the dial too much, you get the wrong sound. So in rehearsal, I started turning the dial too far accidentally. I kept playing a *totally* wrong sound. Instead of bass, I got trumpet. I was getting very agitated over it. It was like my hand had a mind of its own. I told William that I was scared that this was going to happen at the gig. He kept reassuring me that it was not going to happen.

'You have played these songs hundreds of times,' he said reassuringly. 'You will not make a mistake, but even if you did, it would be fine. Just relax.'

I wanted to be as confident as him, as confident as I usually was. I used to be overconfident to the point of arrogance, so this feeling of doubt was foreign and horrible. The thought of turning that damn dial haunted me for days.

On the day of the gig, I practised turning the dial. I practised the same part of the song over and over. I realised that I had to turn the dial with two hands. *Would that look strange?* I thought. *How could I make that look cool instead of awkward?* I was so worried. It was all I could think about.

Hours later, we were at the club playing the sound check. I felt yet another feeling that was a bit foreign to me before a gig. I felt nausea. I was getting myself so nervous over this dial that I felt like vomiting. Friends and family started arriving and I felt even more nervous. Some of them had never seen me perform, and now they were going to see the worst of me. They were going to see a brain-diseased me. I had to get hold of myself. I went into the bathroom to give myself a pep talk. I stared at my reflection in the mirror. *You can do this*, I said mentally. I imagined myself in a boxing ring. My inner coach just shoved the mouth guard in my mouth and said, 'Now get your ass out there, girl!' And so I went.

When the moment of truth came, I acted like a pro. I literally 'acted' like everything was totally cool. As we started playing the song where I switch sounds, I started thinking too much. I was thinking things like, *Oh, this is not bad. Of course you can do this.* Thinking things like this while you're playing can be deadly. I started watching my hands like they were someone else's and I was approving of the playing. Because I had so much subtext in my head, I really did almost forget the music several times. I almost forgot words and notes.

Then the part with the dial got nearer. *Here it comes*, I thought. *Please God, don't let me screw this up. Please!* I started to sweat and my hands started shaking. *Control, Marlo. Control. Smile. Sing. Turn that dial, bitch!* I did it. I did the two-hand turn, slightly awkward, but I did it. Whew! It was such a relief, I felt like screaming. *I can do this!* I shouted inside my head. *I can still do this. The crowd doesn't even know that I have a disease. They can't tell. I am still as good as I ever was; I just need to make tiny adjustments due to my newfound awkward bitch-ness. I can do this!*

The gig went pretty well. There were several mistakes, but none of them were mine! My family and friends who came could not stop commenting on how good I looked and sounded. This was a huge confidence boost for me.

Feeling high from my success at the gig, I continued adjusting to my awkward bitch ways in my everyday life. I was still bumping into things and tripping more than the average person.

One day I saw the lightest-looking little nymph lady enter the store. It was Kate Moss. She was one of the few models I had never seen in person before. I was used to serving this very tall, alien-esque breed of human beings and was thrown off by how different Kate was.

The first thing I realised after greeting her was that I seemed to be looking down at her rather than stretching my neck up as I usually do! I pulled Colin aside while she browsed with a friend she had brought in with her.

'Am I taller than Kate Moss,' I asked him. 'Or has MS really fucked me up?'

'MS fucked you up,' he answered.

At this point Kate had found a classic black tuxedo that she wanted her friend to try on. One of my staff members was serving her.

I continued my line of questioning: 'No, really. I *am* taller, right?'

'Yes,' Colin answered. 'With your wobbly heels you are indeed taller than her! Everyone knows that she is not as tall as other models. That's part of what makes her special. Now go in the fitting room and make sure she's being looked after.'

I headed for the fitting room, where Kate's friend was trying on the tuxedo. The salesperson explained to me that Kate wanted to buy the tuxedo for her friend, perhaps so that she could use her VIP discount. I looked over to Kate. She was cute. She was sweet too. She asked if it was OK that she buys the tuxedo for her friend, and I said that would be fine.

When I asked Kate for her credit card, she opened her gigantic handbag and looked into the chaos that was inside. Suddenly, she squatted down in front of me and turned her handbag upside down. She shook it and spilled the random contents onto the carpet. It took a few shakes before her credit card finally flew out, unaccompanied by a wallet. She handed it up to me. *You're a nutty little one*, I thought. It was during this time that some rumours were starting to surface that she was using cocaine. All I can say is that no cocaine spilled out of her bag!

Two of my staff members turned their heads to either laugh or pretend they did not see Kate on the floor. Her behaviour was indeed odd, but I found it somehow comforting. My behaviour was so odd on an almost hourly basis. With a client like Kate Moss, I did not have to worry about her noticing my awkward bitch ways and thinking I was strange. I wished I had *more* clients like that lovely little nymph.

I was finding a lot of humour in my condition, as many funny things were happening to me. Some people I knew, especially those closest to me at work, also found humour in my condition. They understood that I am someone who finds humour in almost everything, especially that which is otherwise sad. They were not shy about laughing in my face, which sounds cruel, but believe me, it was the best medicine.

One of these people who saw the humour was Dan, our stock manager. You see, I did some awkward bitch things that are typical in people with MS right in front of him.

Dan and I were chatting one day while having lunch. I was eating something called Raspberry Fool, which contains loads of cream. I lifted the spoon to eat a bite, and instead of putting it in my mouth, I smeared it on the side of my face. Remember the problem I had in Paris? It was back. I could not tell where my mouth was once again. Dan's facial expression was priceless.

'What the hell are you doing, Marlo?'

'That's MS,' I said with a smile and a sigh.

We started cracking up laughing. He laughed out of confusion and pure amusement and I laughed out of confusion and pure madness.

Dan saw me do another awkward thing on a different day. I was in the employee's kitchen, making myself coffee. I poured my coffee and walked over to a chair. Dan was watching me walk over to the table and sit down. He looked mildly shocked and severely amused and said, 'Do you not know what just happened?'

'What happened?' I asked. 'Did you do something and I missed it?'

'No,' he replied. '*You* did something and missed it.'

He pointed to the trail of coffee on the floor from the coffeepot to my chair. That was normal enough. Everyone spills things. What was not normal was that I spilt it all over my hands and feet but didn't notice. I did not feel the coffee on my hands, which was a little scary.

'How could you not know that you spilt hot coffee on your hands?' Dan asked.

'I didn't feel it,' I said. I was astonished by it. But before I could ponder it too much, I got distracted by Dan's contagious laughter. He thought it was truly hilarious. I couldn't help but laugh too.

What really amused me, though, was that poor Dan always seemed to be the one to bear witness to my awkward lunchtime problems. At least he always found it comical. Little did he know that his reactions to my troubles actually helped me cope with my life.

Anger Begins

In February, my jubilation over being diagnosed with MS began to wear off. I was feeling less happy and more upset every day. I was entering a new phase of emotions, and it was going to be a rocky road.

People like Dan and Colin, who always laughed with me when I did strange things, were comforting to me. Other people did not react in the same way, though, and I was quickly learning about people's inner weaknesses and inner strengths.

Some people cannot deal with illness. This doesn't make them bad people: it's just the way they are. It is something that no longer upsets me, but back then, it did.

Since my arrival in London, I had been diligent about keeping in touch with friends in the States. From earlier emails, they knew about my eye problems and they had wished me good luck with the doctors. Some of these people, whom I had emailed two months earlier regarding my diagnosis, never emailed me back. Never! I wrote that I had MS and they suddenly fell off the earth. I was hurt.

There were a few people here in London who would avoid me or at least avoid the subject of my health. That also made me angry.

Despite some of the reactions, I continued talking about my diagnosis because I was happy that I was educating people. I was still finding that people didn't know much about MS or had heard of it but did not know exactly what it was. Others had completely wrong ideas about the disease. Several thought it was fatal. Others thought that I would not be able to walk for much longer.

I saw such fear in people's eyes sometimes. I also saw sympathy and pity. That upset me the most. From the days of my diagnosis, I did not want anyone to feel pity for me. I felt that I had a lot going for me and that a stupid little disease like MS was not going to make me any less magnificent. It was not going to make me less talented, less creative, less intelligent, or less anything. *Fuck that*, I thought. *And fuck anyone who pities me.* I still think that, by the way.

On a few occasions, I saw old colleagues on the street (from my hated first job in London), and they asked how my eye was.

'Is your eye better? Did they ever find out what was wrong with it?'

'Oh, yes,' I'd say. 'They found that I have an incurable disease of the brain and nervous system. It's called multiple sclerosis. Have you heard of it?'

I would always say it a bit abruptly, to sort of mindfuck them. I suppose I shocked the hell out of people. They looked like they were sorry that they asked half the time. They were at a loss for words. I guess in retrospect I was angry inside. I would walk away from the conversation feeling a sort of mean satisfaction at letting them down, but I also walked away feeling lonely.

I began to feel a loneliness that I had never quite felt before. I had the support of William, family, and friends like Laura and Colin, but essentially, I was alone with a disease in my brain. Knowing that there is a disease trying to debilitate your body is a lonely thing. No matter who supports you, the ultimate person to help you is yourself.

I am not a particularly religious person, though I am a spiritual one. I believe that God helps those who help themselves, because whatever God is, we are extensions of him. I don't believe in sitting around, waiting for miracles. I wholeheartedly believe in miracles, but I believe that each of us has the power to make a miracle happen ourselves.

Here I was someone who used to have my mom with me when I went to the doctor for a sore throat. Now I was living in a foreign country, with a debilitating disease in my brain, but going to the doctor by myself. Each time I had insisted that William didn't come to doctor appointments, I ended up in waiting rooms feeling alone. I never told him that, because he would never let me go by myself again.

I somehow felt that I *needed* to go alone. I *needed* to feel that way. In all the weeks of learning about other people, I was learning about the most important person of all: myself. I was just starting to learn that I had an inner strength that up until then, I never needed to discover. I was also learning that I had dark places inside me, and at that time, I was slowly sliding down into them.

Some frightening things started to happen to me. Even I couldn't laugh during these times. For example, one day at work, out of nowhere, I had a problem with my speech. I was very tired that day. I was on the selling floor sorting out new merchandise, when a colleague came to ask me a question. I was about to answer him, but when I opened my mouth, nothing came out. For a split second, I could not make my lips form the word. There was some kind of delay in my speech.

I tried to smile and make a sound as if I were saying, 'uh.' I can't be sure that a sound actually came out. I pretended to be thinking about his question, while I scratched my lip to relieve a pretend itch. That bought me a little more time. Because of years of stage experience, I can think quickly on my feet. It's called improvisation, you know?

I'm sure the delay of my words was just a few seconds, but it felt like hours. My palms began sweating in those few seconds. When the words finally did come out, I looked at him fervently to see his reaction. I searched him to see if he knew what had just happened. He just said something like, 'Thanks! See you later!' and popped off.

He was completely oblivious to what had happened. I felt relieved for that, but I was upset. I felt my heart sink into my stomach. *Another problem to add to the list*, I thought. *I can't have this. I can't allow this to happen. The Gemini's mouth can barely keep up with the brain's ideas as it is. I cannot have a speech problem on top of it.*

The speech delay happened two or three more times during the course of the day. Each time it happened, I broke into a small sweat, wondering what the hell was happening to me and worrying that people would notice. I kept trying to do what I did earlier in the day, which was to pretend I was thinking. This cover–up of the problem worked like a charm. No one seemed to notice!

On another workday, I started to get the feeling of bubbles in my head again. Ironically, I was carrying a tray of three glasses of bubbly to clients in the fitting room. As I got near them, my hands just tilted and I dropped the whole tray. The champagne glasses made such a loud noise as they smashed on the marble floor! Colleagues came rushing out of every direction.

'Are you OK, Marlo?'

'Yes, only the champagne was hurt,' I answered, trying to make light of the embarrassing situation.

Hours later, celebrity Sharon Osbourne came in with her personal assistant.

'Hello!' I said to both of them and went running for cover. Usually, a manager would serve a VIP. In fact, I had helped Sharon a few times before, but I just wasn't up for it. I got one of my salesgirls to assist her, though she was a little nervous because it was a celebrity.

'Don't worry,' I told her. 'Sharon is a lovely lady. She pretty much knows what she likes and she's fun. Maybe show her these,' I suggested, pulling out a cashmere cardigan set. 'I'll be hiding in the stockroom if you need my support, OK?'

The bubbles in my head became more explosive. I tried to ignore the feeling by concentrating on work. I tried organising some shoe boxes. As I walked through the aisles, I started to feel very shaky. It was as if I was walking on mushy ground. Everything felt out of the ordinary. I felt like I was on the brink of becoming completely confused. I had to concentrate very hard on staying in reality.

I ended up getting so overwhelmed with dizziness that a member of my staff, Antonello, had to put his arms around me and sit me down in a chair. The colour drained from my face.

'You're the colour of paper,' he said, looking slightly frightened. 'Should I call someone?'

'No,' I answered, 'I'll be fine in a minute.'

'Sharon's buying the cardigan set!' the salesgirl said, coming in to find shoes for her.

'Ex-cel-lent' I answered, in a weak voice.

'Are you OK?' she asked.

'She'll be all right,' Antonello answered.

He rubbed my back and said, 'My poor manager is falling to pieces.'

'I'm still fabulous,' I said, starting to cry. 'I'm still amazing. You know that, right?'

Antonello smiled. 'Of course you are amazing. You are the beautiful Marlo.'

'I'm sorry for all this,' I said, referring to both my present condition and getting MS in general.

'You have nothing to be sorry about. I just want you to take care of yourself. Stop trying to do too many things. You are not helping yourself.'

I knew he was right, but at that point, the thought of slowing down made me too sad. I tried to stretch myself too thin. I wanted to overcompensate for having an illness. I wanted to be Supergirl, no matter what the cost. I thought that if I made myself run at high speed, the MS would not be able to keep up.

'When do you see the neurologist?' Antonello asked.

'Soon,' I answered. 'Soon.'

I didn't want to think about that subject. I had been waiting for over a month just to hear from the neurologist. I rang the hospital so many times during that month, only to find out that referrals got lost and secretaries did not communicate with each other. I finally wrote a letter to the doctor myself, which I believe is why I got the appointment as quickly as I did.

The appointment was set for the second week of February (that was two months after my diagnosis at Moorfields Eye Hospital). I did not think that was acceptable, as I wanted to get on disease-modifying drugs straight away. Some people at work assured me that it was a quick appointment, compared to the usual waiting periods in England. One woman told me her husband had to wait almost one year for a brain scan! Even though it was clearly better than how long others have waited, I did not think that it was good enough. If I lived back in New York, I would have been seen the week after diagnosis, or maybe even days after! But now, what choice did I have? If I wanted the service I received back home, then I would just have to go back home. So instead, I stayed and dealt with it.

The pressure from my family to come home was gaining momentum. There were many medical articles at the time stating that for people diagnosed with MS, the sooner they get on disease-modifying drugs, the better their prognosis. My sisters kept reminding me of this. My mom was praying even more than usual (always a sure sign that things are bad).

I assured them I would be given the disease-modifying drugs at my doctor's appointment or maybe the day after at the latest. I told them that by the time I rang them after the appointment, I probably would have taken my first injection. I wasn't just saying all that. I assumed that was what was going to happen.

The 9th of February came and William and I finally met with the neurologist, Dr. Palmer. I had already heard about this man's great reputation. When I was in one of the many waiting rooms at Moorfields Eye Hospital, I overheard patients talking about how good he was.

He brought us into his office and began looking over the notes that the Mister from Moorfields Eye Hospital had written. He asked me questions about my symptoms and gave me a neurological exam. The exam included laying me down and poking my legs, feet, arms, hands, face, and abdomen with a little stick, to see if I had feeling. After this, he tested the same areas with a piece of cotton wool.

From this, I realised that I had no feeling on the right side of my abdomen. I actually had not noticed this until the exam. He looked at my eyes with a small torch. I had to follow his torch with my eyes as he glided it from side to side. He had me touch my finger to his finger and then to my nose. Then I had to perform this faster.

After the physical exam, we all sat down and briefly discussed MS. The doctor said something to me like, 'Well, you definitely have MS and I can see that you have done quite a lot of research on it, so you know what it involves.'

I hadn't realised that the doctors at Moorfields did not have the last word on my diagnosis. *This* doctor had the last word, and yes, I had MS. It was quite anticlimactic, in fact. William and I looked at each other in disbelief. *Yes, and? So now what?*

I asked him many questions about the disease-modifying drugs that were available, based on research I had done. He did not tell me which drug he thought would be best for me. He said that it would ultimately be my decision. I told him that I wanted to be put on the interferons straight away, and he said that he would refer me to the MS nurses at the hospital.

'The MS nurses are the people who MS patients usually have the most contact with,' he said. 'The nurses are the ones who start you on the drug and teach you how to inject, and so on.'

That was all he said. That was the visit I had waited so long for. I waited two months to hear again that I had MS. Fabulous.

'Oh my God,' I said to William when we left the office.

'I don't believe it,' he answered, shaking his head. 'What the hell was this appointment for?'

'What am I going to tell my mom?' I asked him rhetorically. 'She is going to flip out! My sisters will go mad!'

'I don't believe it,' he repeated. 'What should we do now?'

'Eat, of course,' I answered. 'We need comfort.'

We went to a nearby sandwich shop, where we witnessed an Italian man behind the counter verbally abusing his staff and the customers.

'Whadda you want?' he shouted at us.

'He's a sandwich Nazi,' William whispered.

'Shhh,' I said. 'He'll slap us.'

We sat down with our sun-dried tomato sandwiches and cups of tea, discussing the disappointing doctor's visit. We started laughing watching the abusive man interact with what we were sure were loyal customers.

'Imagine if I told him the tomatoes in my sandwich are not fresh,' William joked. 'He'd say, *I'll show you a fuckin' fresh tomato, you sonna ma bitch!'*

We got hysterical laughing. We somehow found comfort in the abusive man's sandwich shop. The sandwiches were in fact, delicious. In the future, we too would become loyal customers.

Hours later, I was on the phone with my family.

'What happened?' my mom asked.

'Not a whole lot,' was my response.

'What? This is terrible,' she said. 'It's outrageous!' One by one, my sisters got on the phone to tell me the same thing.

'You'd better come home,' was everyone's response. 'You are obviously not getting the treatment that you need over there. You must come home.'

They told me about a new drug in the United States called Tysabri or Natalizumab, as it was called in Europe. It was getting press all over the television and newspapers. Talk show hosts like Larry King were bringing on famous people who have MS. Some of these celebs said that they were going to start taking Tysabri soon.

This drug was very different from the interferons. First, it was said to perhaps slow the disease down by 60 per cent! This was quite an improvement. Second, it was taken intravenously once a month.

'Wow,' I said in a defeated low voice. 'That is a huge difference from the other drugs, the drugs that I am not even on yet. Maybe I will have to move back to the States, after all.'

I wondered why the drug was available in the States and not in the UK. My mind was an overture of questions: a thick Wagnerian overture, not a light and airy Mozart one.

What drug will I take? Are these drugs even safe? Should I be taking this Tysabri? Is there a risk in taking this drug? Is there a medical reason why it is not approved in the UK? Are doctors in the States better qualified to treat MS? Am I making a huge mistake staying here?

My questions were endless.

In an effort to answer my own questions, I again immersed myself in Internet research. I was confused as to why the doctor did not recommend one drug over the other. I was trying to decide which one I would want to take, and the choice was not easy. There seemed to be many side effects. For example, the beta interferons all seemed to cause flu-like symptoms in most people. Some caused skin irritation. They all seemed to do the same thing, though, so what was the difference? I was getting more confused.

Then, I found a great website that helps you decide what drugs would be right for you. On this particular website, I took a forty minute test to see what drug would suit my lifestyle. I took the test twice and came up with two different answers at the end. Despite the two different answers, I found it helpful. It did narrow down my possibilities from four drugs to two.

I started to research more on Tysabri. I found out that it was not approved in the UK yet, because the National Institute for Health and Clinical Excellence (NICE), an independent organisation that provides guidance to the NHS, did not think that enough tests had been done to prove its safety and cost-effectiveness. It had to be proven to be cost effective, since medicine here is socialised.

I kept digging further and further though articles. It was through my rigorous Internet surfing that I discovered the truths about these drugs, politics, and money in the UK. It was not pretty.

As any of us know these days, where there are drugs to be had (and I mean legal drugs in this case), there is money to be made. But what happens if there is money to be *lost?* What then? Let me explain.

The disease-modifying drugs are expensive. They can cost anywhere from £8,000 to £18,000 a year. In the States, where the drugs have been licensed for a longer period of time, this is not much of a problem, if you have health insurance. Insurance companies pay for most of it. If you don't have health insurance, though, you are either screwed or you have to be a little savvy and do your research. Provided that you are a

US resident, many drug companies will sponsor your drug treatment! My sister Lorraine found that out for me. Her friend's sister had MS and no health insurance. She was able to get on one of the beta interferons through a charity run by the drug company itself.

In the UK, however, the drugs are issued under what is called a 'risk sharing' program. Because the long-term effects of the drugs had not been proven, paying for them is a risk to the payer. So, the NHS and the drug companies have made a risk-sharing deal. They agree that the NHS will foot the bills, but if in ten years, the drugs prove ineffective to the patients taking them, the drug companies will pay for the bills. I know it sounds complicated, and if I were you, I would read this paragraph a few times.

It gets more interesting though. I started to realise that not everyone who had MS in the UK was able to get on the drugs. In the UK, these drugs are mainly used for people with the relapsing-remitting form of MS, like me. There were definitive criteria that a patient had to meet.

The first was that you had to have relapsing-remitting multiple sclerosis. Second, you had to be able to walk 100 feet without assistance.

What the hell is this? I thought. *If you can't walk 100 feet on the day of your test, they tell you, sorry, no drugs for you?* Of the people who meet these criteria, the NHS was allowing people to get the drug as part of a lottery. I could not believe my eyes when I read about this.

'A fucking lottery!' I screamed to the computer screen. In other words, if you were lucky enough to win, you could be treated. Was this a game? I did not understand.

I started finding documentation on this subject all over the Internet. On one popular MS site, you could click on a button that linked to a recording of the cries of protesters who marched in London for people to get fair access to the disease-modifying drugs. My heart sank listening to them. There were many pictures of people carrying signs reading '2 YEARS AND STILL WAITING'. *Two years? People with MS, people like me, were waiting for two years and more to receive the help that they were entitled to?* I was sobbing my heart out looking at these people suffering. Here I was getting upset because I had waited two months!

I could not understand how a kingdom as wealthy as this one was letting so many of its people down. Apparently, the NICE committee members were the ones who made all these decisions. I was so angry with them. I was also scared that if I waited too long, I would not be able to walk without assistance.

In the coming days, I made an effort not to worry, but it was futile. I could not stop thinking about getting on the interferons. I became obsessed with it. My family tried to reason with me, insisting that I move back home. I did not want to move back home because I had a disease that was not being treated here. *That would make me a failure,* I thought. I could imagine people saying, 'How was London. You got tired of it?'

'No, I acquired an incurable disease, so here I am back in New York. Tra la la!'

No way could I let that happen. I came to London to live here for some time. I came to make my mark, and my own band was not even formed yet! I had not played a Marlo show in one whole year, and now I was getting depressed. I was not moving back.

I waited one week after seeing Dr. Palmer for an MS nurse to contact me and when one didn't, I rang the hospital, and let me tell you, I was in a rage. I was at work when I made the phone call. The nurse whom I spoke to had my referral, which was a relief. However, the relief wore off when she explained to me that I could not get the beta interferons at the National Hospital because I lived in a postal code that this hospital didn't serve. She told me I would have to be referred to another hospital closer to where I lived. She seemed to be saying that I could still attend the clinics at the National Hospital, but because of the risk sharing program, I would need to get the interferons from the hospital in my postcode. My eyes filled with tears. I asked her how long she thought it would take from this point to get on them.

She said, 'Probably two to three months.' I thought I would have a mental breakdown right there on the phone.

'What if I pay for the drugs myself?' I asked her. I thought about perhaps taking out a loan or raising money somehow.

'That would not be possible,' she said.

I hung up feeling confused and emotionally drained. I rang her back a few times, hounding her with more questions. Who was my neurologist now? I don't have one? Where and when will I finally be treated? Am I treated at one hospital? Or two? Or none?

I kept telling her, 'I don't understand what you are saying!' I felt so alone. I felt exhausted too. This was partly from frustration and partly from the fact that another relapse was coming on.

Shit

ઈ૦

Is it inappropriate to tell your boss that you are running late due to the fact that you've just had to wipe your ass twenty to thirty times and it took longer than expected? This was the new situation I found myself in.

For one solid week, I would get to my front door to leave for work in the morning and then almost crap my pants. After the actual defecation, which took ages, I would wipe my bum over and over and over. The stool was a bit loose, hence the arduous task of wiping.

It was a bad feeling. I tried to laugh, and well, I did laugh, at first. I was late every single day that week. I told my boss that I was having some 'problems' in the mornings.

This little problem happened at night too. I could not deal with it very well. I started having temper tantrums on the toilet. William had to endure the tantrums. I would slump over the toilet screaming at the top of my lungs, 'How many times can a human being wipe their fucking ass before the paper is clean? How many fucking times?' I was roaring!

William laughed at first, but as this got to be a nightly thing, the humour kind of died. My bum was sore for a couple of weeks, and so were William's ears.

The crapping was also more frequent than what I would consider normal. I worked with several people who, for various reasons, were often blocked, and a good shit was an event for them. I wished that was my case, because I seemed to go four times a day that week.

One evening towards the end of the week, I was stuck in the ladies' toilet at the end of a workday. The employee toilet was attached to the locker room where we girls all changed. I sat there trying to shit quietly, as everyone left one by one. As was usual that week, I wiped and flushed and wiped and flushed (you get the idea).

This is really sucking, I thought. When I finally finished, I realised that the lights of the store were turned off. My heart sank to my stomach! *Someone forgot I was here and locked me in!*

I ran through a hallway in the darkness and made my way up the same staircase that I had stumbled up half blind in the previous weeks! I got to the front door of the store just in time to see Simon putting down the security gate outside.

I shouted, 'Simon!'

He looked at me and screamed. 'Ah! Oh my God!'

We started laughing as he let me out and apologised. *My ass is really getting me into bad situations,* I thought.

It was during this 'bad ass' time, at the end of February, that I started to know a suffering that I had never known. It began with a few nights of bad sleep. I would get into bed, and just as my body started to relax, I would feel a tingle in the bottom of my foot. The tingle was a tightening of the muscle. It would not let up and kept me up for most of the night. Each night the feeling got a little tighter.

Then, without warning, the situation worsened. It was probably the fourth night, when the tingle in my foot started to creep up the back of my leg to the knee. The tingling became a prelude for a pain that became my nightly torturous companion. The tightening had become a feeling of ripping and burning. I felt like my leg muscle was being ripped apart and twisted.

After a few more nights, the pains began to sneak into the other foot and leg as well. In the States, the term 'charley horse' is used when your foot cramps underneath it and up into the back of your leg. This was like a double charley horse orchestrated by the devil himself.

I took several different types of painkillers, and none of them worked. I put ice on my legs; that didn't work. I put heat on them; that didn't work. For the most part, I did not fall asleep during all of this. If I did get to sleep, the pain would wake me up a while later.

Each night, the pain would reach new levels of intensity. The level of pain that I had described as 'very bad' in the first week, later reached a level of excruciating. It was a level of pain that I did not imagine existed without getting shot or stabbed. The severe cramps not only went down the back of my legs, and under my feet, but also went into my toes. I looked down at my toes at one point, and I could actually see them jumping and stretching all by themselves! They were in spasm.

It became pure torture. For three solid weeks, every night I would get in bed and pray, 'Please God let me sleep tonight.' Just as I would start to doze off, I would feel the tingles, and then the pain, worsening deeper and deeper into the land of excruciation. I would start gasping from it. At the height of each spasm, I could not breathe.

This severe pain would switch on and off for hours. It would suddenly stop, and I had a few minutes to rest, catch my breath, and wipe the tears that had made pools in my ears. Then the cramping would start all over again.

Sometimes I would imagine myself on a torture rack in some medieval time. In this fantasy, each of my toes was stabbed with jagged hooks that were attached to ropes. Those ropes were tied to a big wheel. That wheel was then turned, stretching my toes and legs to the point of almost breaking the wheel.

Whilst this went on, someone took more hooks and forced them into the bottoms of my feet. They twisted and turned the hooks whilst the wheel turned. My imaginative mind tried to come up with a story to accompany the agony I was in. Some imagination.

At certain moments of the misery, I would start laughing hysterically out of madness. I began wishing that we lived on a higher floor, so that I could jump out the window. Killing myself started to look like a pleasant escape from the hell I was in.

For those three weeks I was up every single night. Sadly, William could not sleep either. I suggested that I sleep on the sofa, but he would not hear of it. He insisted that I stay in the bed with him so that he could comfort me. He would massage my feet and legs when the cramps initially started each night. Then he would intermittently fall in and out of sleep through the night. I would think about how William would be wrecked in the morning. He kept saying that he was fine, and that he could still get enough sleep. The purple rings under his eyes told me another story, though.

I, for one, was becoming overwhelmingly exhausted from lack of sleep and pain. Each morning I would sit on a chair to put my trousers on. I was so tired; I could not balance myself standing. I would put one leg in my trousers, then close my eyes and sleep for a minute. Then I would put the other leg in.

I just want to die, I kept thinking. I would sometimes compose a suicide note in my head: *Dear William, I love you more than life itself. You are everything to me. But, I cannot live in this pain anymore. Please understand and please tell my mom and my sisters how much I love them and that I am so sorry....*

I was finding my job to be extremely difficult, almost impossible. I could barely keep my eyes open; plus the cramps were occurring on a milder scale during the day too. Sometimes, a cramp would come on, and I would limp for a few minutes. Then it would pass. Between the pains and the exhaustion, I constantly felt like vomiting.

I made a daily habit of going into the employee bathroom to slump over the toilet and rest my head on the loo roll. I would close my eyes and pretend my head was resting comfortably on a little cloud. I could actually doze off for a few minutes in that position. Then I would open my eyes and look down at my feet.

I watched the tips of my beautiful Yves Saint Laurent shoes move as my toes would spasm out of control inside them.

I would try to encourage myself in the cubicle.

'You will be fine, Marlo,' I'd say in a whisper. 'Now get your ass off this toilet bowl and get out there!'

I did not know at the time that what was happening was another relapse. I did not understand what I was experiencing, and I did not know whom to call. I felt alone and very unwell. At that point, it was the worst sickness I had ever felt in my life.

One morning, a few weeks into the relapse, it all came to a head while I was at work. I started to get a dreaded bladder infection and I was out of my stash of antibiotics. I noticed it when passing urine was slightly difficult and I felt a twinge of pain in my abdomen. Then the cramping in my legs got unusually bad for daytime hours. By midday, I turned the colour of chalk. I actually felt crazy. I developed a severe pain in my bladder to accompany the escalating cramps in my legs and feet. I was about to pass out.

I went up to Simon to tell him I felt ill, and before I could get the words out, he knew.

'Sit down!' he ordered.

My co-workers got me a chair and water, while Simon rang a taxi for me. I was embarrassed and in so much pain. I started crying. I felt so sick and depressed. Whilst I waited for the cab, I rang my general practitioner (GP). He was out of the office, but by some mistake of his receptionist, I was connected straight to his mobile phone. He was actually driving in his car!

I was expecting the receptionist to answer.

'Hello?' I heard a man's voice say.

'Sorry,' I answered. 'I have the wrong number; I meant to ring a surgery.' I started to hang up. With the phone almost on the receiver, I heard his voice come blaring through the phone.

'This *is* the surgery!' he shouted.

I put the phone back up to my ear. 'Doctor?' I asked. 'Is that you?'

'Yes,' he answered. 'Who is this?'

'I'm your patient, Marlo Parmelee. I have a bladder infection and I also have MS, and I am *so* sick!' I was ranting on for so long, I am not sure what else I said to him.

He told me that he could not see me because the office was shut. I asked, 'Where do I go?' Once again I felt like there was no one in the medical field who could take care of me. Then a miracle happened. He must have heard the desperation in my voice. He asked if I had bladder infections before. I told him I did, and explained what medication I had always taken. He told me that he would call a prescription in to the pharmacy in my town, and that I could go immediately to pick it up. I was so relieved!

The cab ride home was horrible. I was doubling up in pain from the bladder and the legs. I thought I was going to urinate on the seat. I kept praying that I wouldn't. I was sweating profusely and shaking out of control. My teeth were chattering louder than the engine of the car. I later wondered if the taxi driver thought I was someone coming down off of heroin. At the time, I could care less what he thought. I asked him to take me to the pharmacy before taking me home.

When I went into the pharmacy, I gave the pharmacist my name and said that the doctor had just called in my prescription.

'No one rang,' he said.

'That can't be,' I shrieked. 'I just spoke to him!' I did not have a mobile phone with me, and I had left the doctor's number at work. I had no choice but to go home and ring from there.

I ran out in a rage. I got back into the taxi and went home. When I got in my door, I ran to the bathroom. I was in agony. I was urinating thick blood, as I always did from these infections. I could barely leave the toilet to get to the phone. I was so annoyed at myself for not buying a cordless phone the year before. Then I could have phoned from the toilet.

I raced to the phone and rang the doctor in his car again. He told me that he pulled over to ring the pharmacy but they were not answering. I asked could he ring again, but he told me to ring them and tell *them* to ring *him.* What a nightmare! I just wanted the damn antibiotics!

I rang the pharmacist and he refused to ring the doctor, saying that usually the doctor rings him. I became quite desperate. 'Please ring him! He is driving and cannot pull over to dial your number again! He already tried to ring you and I am *very, very* sick!' My voice was shaking as it got louder. I sounded like someone on the edge. I *was* someone on the edge.

Then the pharmacist agreed to do it. I ran back to the toilet to pee more painful blood. I came back to the phone and rang the pharmacist again to make sure he now had the prescription. He did. I ran back to the toilet again. I was not sure how I would get down to the pharmacy. It was three bus stops away. I was bent over in pain, and I did not think that holding my bladder was possible. I did one last agonizing pee, stuffed a wad of loo paper in my panties, and bolted for the door.

Waiting minutes for the bus seemed like hours. I prayed to my dad, who had died in 1999.

'Please, Dad, get me through this. Please help me do this.'

When the bus came, I was so bent over that I was close to a crawling position. Two elderly ladies cut me off to get in front of me on the queue. They were not looking at me until we all boarded. When they realised the condition I was in, one of them offered me her seat. I ignored her and went to the back of the bus. I could not sit down anyway. Between the bladder pain and the relentless leg cramping, I was in brutal agony.

The bus stopped in front of the pharmacy. Inside, I practically shouted my name to the woman behind the counter. When she got my prescription, I threw the money in front of her. The woman started slowly putting the pills in a bag.

'No bag!' I screamed. She was looking at me like I was a lunatic. I thought I would vomit on her, piss myself, or pass out on the floor. I did not care if I did all three.

I ran out of there and darted into the store next door to buy juice. I swallowed the pills there in the store. I could not wait to get home. The bus ride back home was much like the journey there: pure agony. My head was spinning. I prayed to my dad the whole way back as well and I believe that is the reason I did not pass out. I focused on him so intensely that it kept my mind alert. By the time I got back home, I had only peed in my pants a little. That was quite a feat!

The medication took effect within the hour. It had been another exhausting day of MS-related problems. I felt so low and I was getting so tired of feeling sick. I did not think that I could take much more.

Hopelessness

&

That night I noticed another wacky symptom of MS. I was leaning over to zip up my jeans, when a weird thing happened. As I leaned my head forward (chin towards chest), I got a feeling of a *zap* in my foot. It was not a bad feeling. It was a beautiful bolt of electricity. It tickled, actually. It was the first time I had felt something good in a while. I kept putting my chin to my chest to get the feeling again.

'I know what this is,' I said to William, as I continued putting my chin to my chest. 'I've read about this. It's called L'Hermitte's sign.'

William got on the Internet and read from one of the MS websites.

'It's named after the man who discovered it. It is common in MS. An electrical impulse goes down the spine and possibly the legs when the person brings his or her head forward.'

'Why does it happen?' I asked.

William read on. 'It says that it's from lesions on the spinal cord.'

'So now they have spread to my spine,' I said. 'Abigail and her bastard friends are multiplying.'

The idea of the disease's progression was scary for me. I did not want to think of the little fuckers scarring my spine too. I tried to just amuse myself with the zap feeling.

'I think you should stop doing that,' William said.

He was afraid that I would make things worse if I continued to lean my head forward over and over.

'I can't stop,' I said, leaning my head forward again. 'I like this feeling. It's the first good feeling I have had in weeks.'

'You *must* stop!' he begged. 'It can't be good for you!'

I think he was also tired of hearing me say 'Whooh!' every single time I did it.

The next day, I went to see the GP who got me the antibiotics. He was only prepared to talk about the bladder infection and send me away quickly. He didn't mention the fact that I had MS, so I mentioned it.

'Who told you that?' he asked, looking confused.

I was shocked by this response. 'Uh....
the neurologist at the National Neurological
Hospital. Didn't they send you my notes?'

'They didn't send me any notes!' he said
angrily.

'Well, don't you have the notes from
Moorfields Eye Hospital saying that I have
MS?'

'No! The last notes that they sent me say
that you are having an MRI and then that was
it.'

'OK, well I don't know what to say. I don't
even know where I'm supposed to go to be
treated,' I said.

'They should have sent me the notes so that
I can refer you to a neurologist in this area.
You must see someone in the proper postcode!
I am going to refer you to Dr. Smith, who is an
excellent neurologist at Wandsworth Hospital.
As soon as you leave my office, I am going to
ring him myself!'

He was visibly upset, which I thought was
great for my case. He seemed to be on my
side. Now I felt hopeful that I could get on the
interferons sooner than later.

'This is unbelievable!' he continued. 'You
can't treat people like this. You can't tell
someone they are diagnosed with MS, and then
send them away.'

'Right on!' I wanted to shout. I left the
office feeling relieved that I would now get
an appointment with this great doctor at

Wandsworth Hospital and things would start to happen!

To make a long story short, I never got to see the great doctor at Wandsworth Hospital. When I hadn't heard from his office, I rang them and found out that I was never referred to him.

How can that be? My GP was so angry; he was ringing him the minute I left the office.

I rang my GP to find out who was lying, him or the hospital. I found out it was him!

'I rang Dr. Smith and he was not there,' he said. 'My secretary mailed him a referral and mailed you a copy too. Didn't you get it?'

'No,' I answered. 'I did not get any copy of a referral.'

'I will send another one and send you another copy. In a few days, I suggest you ring Dr. Smith again.'

So, I did just that. Again, I did not receive a copy of a referral and again the secretary of Dr. Smith had never heard of me. She asked me what it was that I was referred for. I told her that I had MS, and she told me that Dr. Smith does not work with patients with MS. His specialty was something else. My heart sank once more.

That week I was back and forth on the phone with four different doctors and three different hospitals. My GP started accusing me of changing my address, saying that was why the referrals got lost. I hadn't changed my address! It was getting so stupid. No one had answers for me and my own doctor was lying. I was getting nowhere.

I was so fed up, sick, and depressed that I started throwing tantrums in our flat. I was hitting rock bottom. William would come home from work and find the place ransacked and me crying in a ball in the corner of the room.

He would try to comfort me. My reaction to him was usually one of throwing myself on the bed, pounding my fists on the pillows, screaming.

'Why me? Why? Why? Why?' I shouted over and over.

I smashed cups and plates and put holes in the walls.

William had the daunting task of trying to calm me down. 'Marlo, everything will be OK.'

'Don't tell me everything is going to be OK!' I would roar. 'I am in so much fucking pain! None of the painkillers have helped me! I want to jump off the fucking roof! Do you understand? I want to kill myself! I want to die! I want to fucking die! Why can't this country help me? What the hell is wrong with these people? Why the hell does it have to be so hard? I am so tired. I have never been so tired....'

We were both completely drained at that point. I started phoning my mom and crying to her. I would rant and rave about how I was not getting treatment in the UK, and I would have to come home.

Then she would say, 'Now you are thinking clearly! You have to come back to the States.'

'Yes,' I would say. 'I am coming back.'

Hours later, I would ring her back and say, 'No, I am not coming back.' I did this to my sisters as well. It got to the point where everyone was getting fed up.

'You are all over the place,' Lisa said. 'One minute you're up, the next you're down. You're moving back. You're *not* moving back!'

'I know,' I muttered.

'If you were home, you would be on beta interferons already, and you would be getting steroid treatment for this relapse that you are in.'

'You think this is a relapse?' I asked, sniffling.

'All this pain you have, these sound like spasms. To me, this sounds like a relapse. I think you need steroids, but the neurologist needs to tell you all this.'

My mom got on the phone next. 'Just relax and the answer will come to you,' she advised.

Well I wasn't relaxing and the answer wasn't coming. William wondered if he should start looking for a job in New York.

'What do you want to do?' he kept asking. Finally he said, 'That's it. We are moving back home! That is where you can get the best health care. It's over. We are moving back and I don't want to hear another word about it!'

I decided he was right. At that point, there was nothing left to do but go back to the States. I was beaten down. I felt that I was finished fighting for every little appointment. Socialised medicine of course has its upsides, like not having to worry about paying a doctor's bill when you have the flu. But I was seeing the downside: the major downside.

∞

I was crying as I started packing up my knick-knacks in bubble wrap. I couldn't stop thinking of all the gigs I hadn't played yet, all the plans I had not finished or hadn't even started yet. I thought of the friendships I had made, including my new friendship with Magdalara. I wanted to know more about her. I felt that we had met for a reason, and if I left, I would never find out what that reason was. I knew I belonged here in London and yet I was packing to leave.

My mom and sisters were ecstatic when I told them that my new 'final, final' decision was to move back home. They were already helping me research what doctors to contact when I came home. They were all on the Internet. They were calling friends who had friends with MS and asking them where they go for treatment. They had all kinds of leads for me.

They were happy finding out everything for the baby of the family. They could tell I was not happy with the thought of moving home, though. They all felt sad that I was not that happy about it. I did miss them badly, but moving back felt wrong. Leaving London felt wrong. Leaving my job felt wrong. It *all* felt wrong.

I still have the resignation letter I wrote to Simon saved on my computer. When I typed it up, I could barely see because I was crying so hard. I kept wiping my face and the keyboard.

I wrote in the letter how I was so sorry to have to leave a job that I loved. I felt at that point, because I was not getting rapid enough help from the NHS, that I was jeopardising my health. I explained how I would need to move back to the States, where I could get the kind of care I needed. It was very sad.

I brought the letter into work the next day. I kept it in my pocket for the entire morning. Everything was business as usual, but I felt like I was about to drop a bomb. I did not want to give Simon the letter. I did not want to leave London, especially for this reason.

I tried to give the letter to him several times, but I could not bring myself to take it out. At one point I told him I needed to speak to him, and instead of giving him the letter, I came up with some lame reason about something work related. I started to feel nauseous. My heart was in my stomach.

Finally, in the afternoon, I realised I had to get it over with. I took Simon aside and said, 'I don't want to give you this.' The letter was shaking in my hand. He looked at it and knew straight away what it was.

'If it's your resignation, then I don't want to take it,' he said.

Both of us started to well up with tears.

'Is there anything we can do so that you don't have to go? I'm gutted,' he said. We talked about it for a few minutes, but found it too difficult to continue the conversation.

We both spent the rest of the day completely depressed. Every time we saw each other on the shop floor, we would say something like, 'I am devastated,' or 'I'm pretending it's not real.' I kept trying to smile, but my heart was breaking inside. *This is insanity,* I thought. *It's worse than a damn break-up.* It didn't feel right.

On the way home that night, I felt like my world was crashing. I looked at people on the pavement, walking to wherever they were going. *You don't have MS,* I thought. *You don't have to leave a city you love because the NHS can't deal with your fucking illness! Why can't I be one of these other people? Why does this have to be my fucking reality? I came here to live a dream. Why can't I live it? Because some stupid disease is trying to stop me? What happened to the Marlo I used to be? She was healthy and unstoppable. Where did she go?*

I took a bus home that night. I started sobbing uncontrollably as I sat by a window. My tissues turned to wet balls. I kept my head down, trying to conceal my tears. My desperate monologue of *Why me?* continued in my head. Then the strangest thing happened....

Hope
೮೧

I lifted my head to look out the window. At the moment I looked out, I saw black graffiti on a white wall in gigantic letters. It read 'DON'T GO'.

My mouth dropped open as I sat straight up in my seat. The hair on the back of my neck stood up. I can't describe the feeling accurately. I had a profound moment of clarity.

What was even weirder was that the words read in the direction that the bus was going. I was reading from right to left. If you read them from the other direction, from left to right, you would have seen 'GO DON'T'. I should mention that the bus was travelling at turtle speed, and I had a good deal of time to stare at the words.

My tears stopped flowing and my pity party came to an abrupt halt. Suddenly my mind cleared for the first time in ages. I got off the bus knowing for certain that I could not leave London. Abigail and her friends could fuck themselves. If staying meant jeopardising my health, then I would jeopardise it.

When I got home, I was exuberant. I explained to William what had happened on the bus. I was talking so fast, I had to repeat myself a few times. He got very emotional. He said that we would stay if I wanted to stay or go if I wanted to go. He did not care anymore. It was too much of an emotional roller coaster.

I rang Simon on his mobile. He was in a pub telling his friend about my resignation.

'I'm just talking about you,' he said. 'I had to have a drink.'

'Simon, I've changed my mind. I am not leaving London. I can't do it. I have never been so miserable about anything in my life. I want to take back my resignation.'

He was stunned. 'Are you sure? What changed?' I am sure that he was wary that I would change my mind back the next day, but I assured him that this was my final decision. I explained why I had to stay. I was in such high spirits, I was almost screaming into the phone.

The next day, Simon looked at me and smiled.

'I'm so happy,' he said. 'I was really sick over it yesterday.'

'So was I,' I said. He handed me the letter I had given to him the previous day. I put it in the rubbish bin and smiled.

There is an expression, 'The writing is on the wall.' For me it was literal and it was mind blowing. In later days, I looked to see the words again but did not know where the bus had been when I saw it. William later saw the writing near Stockwell station and pointed it out to me. It was then painted over in white a few days later.

Over the next couple of weeks, I started to recover from the relapse. This was partially due to the fact that I bribed a friend to give me his leftover oral steroids from an injury he had. When Lisa explained to me that she thought I was in a relapse, I started to understand what was happening to me. When she said that I probably needed steroids, I did some research.

I administered the steroids to myself, according to guidelines I found on the Internet. I decided if I had to be my own doctor, then I would be. If the government was not going to help, then I would help myself. I was no longer going to be a victim. I was becoming proactive. I would do anything it took to make myself better whilst living in London. The reign of the bad shit and sleepless nights was coming to an end.

Oh, the vanity! One night, Carol rang to tell me more about the MS centre she had gone to. She had actually gotten the number of her own centre and another one that was closer to where I lived.

Carol told me about one particular therapy she used to partake in called *hyperbaric oxygen therapy*. Basically, it is a treatment that simulates deep-sea diving. You go through all the motions of diving, with mask on and all, but you are not in water. The oxygen that you breathe through the mask is pure oxygen. When you breathe pure oxygen in a pressurised environment, the oxygen enriches your cells, at a profound rate. She told me that many people with MS have found this therapy quite helpful. They had more energy and felt well. She said it did wonders for her. In fact, she swore by it. The only reason she had to stop was because she had tinnitus (ringing in the ears).

Although I was open to any suggestion, I felt that this type of therapy was probably not for me. I would not go diving in the sea if there were fish to look at, so why would I go diving on land when there are *no* fish to look at? She explained that you sit in a small pod with other MS patients. *Small pod?* I pondered. *The Jacques Cousteau of MS.* This sounded like the stuff that claustrophobic nightmares are made of. *No, this is not for me,* I thought.

Then Carol said one sentence guaranteed to change the mind of a vain little awkward bitch like me: 'When I was doing the oxygen,' she said, 'nobody knew I was doing it, but everyone was telling me I looked years younger.'

She went on to say that people were accusing her of having facial work! Now I was listening. *Hmm,* I thought. *I should give this a chance. After all, Carol has gone through all this trouble to get me these phone numbers. Not to mention, I can perhaps combat the fine lines that can creep around your eyes during times of stress; times like this! Never mind the MS,* I thought. *I can look like a teenager again! How fabulous! Maybe MS had finally given me some kind of fringe benefit instead of suicidal thoughts!* I decided that the oxygen therapy was for me after all.

When I got off the phone with Carol, I started researching hyperbaric oxygen therapy on the Internet. What I found was that many football teams use this therapy for players who are injured. If a footballer sustains an injury like a broken arm, for example, breathing pure oxygen can heal it faster than it would heal on its own. The oxygen speeds up the body's natural healing process.

This can be very costly, though. I was finding prices on US sites that were $15,000 for ten sessions. If this was the price of the treatment, then maybe it wasn't for me. I decided I had better ring the MS centre straight away to find out prices. I did not want to get my hopes up for nothing.

When I rang the centre, I discovered that it offered a lot more than just hyperbaric oxygen treatment. It offered all kinds of alternative therapies for MS, not to mention other diseases. It offered acupuncture, massage, reiki, and reflexology. It sounded like a one-stop spa for MS. It got even better, too. Because the centre was run mostly by charity, there were no high prices to pay! I sound like an infomercial, I know. Each session cost around £8–£14. All you needed was your doctor's consent. How easy. *Now* I was excited! I was going as soon as possible.

Days later, with my doctor's consent in hand, I took two long train rides and a bus to the MS centre in Walthamstow (East London). Walking from the bus stop, I realised that if I was having a bad relapse, I could not travel there alone. It was too far. The first thing I noticed when I walked into the centre was that it looked like a neighbourhood community centre. It was informal and slightly cluttered. The waiting room had a table filled with knick-knacks that were for sale.

The people there were extremely pleasant and made me feel at home straight away, including John, the attendant who showed me around. John explained to me what hyperbaric oxygen was all about. He told me how the premiership footballers use this as a treatment for injuries, just as I had read on the Internet.

He showed me the pod where I would be getting the oxygen. It was like a small silver spaceship sitting in the middle of a room. It had lots of pipes and tubes going in and out of it. It had several small windows that you would expect to see on a little ship. There was a solid-looking hatch door with a wheel on it.

'It can fit about six people, including wheelchairs,' he explained.

I couldn't help but smile when I saw that there were cute paintings of fish and bubbles all over the pod. In fact, there was a whole underwater world painted on it.

'This was painted by a group of volunteer schoolchildren,' he told me.

'It's great,' I said.

Then he asked me, 'What do you hope to get out of this?'

Holding back a naughty grin, I was about to say, 'Eight years off my face,' but I refrained. I told him that I would just like to see if perhaps I felt better. If he only knew my real intentions!

John told me that I would be in the pod with a man called Steve and pointed to a man sitting in another room chatting to someone. I looked in at him and noticed that he had a bandage around his leg but otherwise looked completely healthy. I assumed that he was there for a sporting injury. He was slightly limping when he walked. He looked like a football coach or a ski instructor. I figured his doctor probably sent him there for a speedy recovery.

When the scheduled dive time came, Steve and I entered the pod. A man outside closed the hatch behind us and turned the wheel. *OK, we're now locked in,* I thought. *Here we go, Marlo. You got yourself into this pod business, and you are not getting out.* I gave Steve a little smile.

In a moment of awkward silence, I was dying to turn to him and say, 'So, do you come here often?' I stopped myself.

Steve introduced himself and asked me if I had ever done the oxygen before. He told me that he had done it numerous times and told me what to expect. He explained how the pod would first compress. It made you feel like you were on an airplane that was landing. Steve told me that it was best to swallow at least every thirty seconds, or else too much pressure would build in your ears. He was very informative and I enjoyed listening to him.

The compression took fifteen minutes, so we had plenty of time to chat. He asked me why I was there and I told him that I had MS. He asked me when I was diagnosed, and so on. He seemed to know a lot about MS. I thought he must know a lot of people with MS from coming to this centre.

'Why do *you* come here?' I asked him. 'For your leg?'

He looked surprised by my question. 'I'm here for the same reason as you,' he said. 'I have MS as well.'

I was shocked! 'I thought you were here for a leg injury,' I told him. 'A sports injury!'

He smiled and explained to me that his foot was not lifting off the ground when he tried to walk. To compensate for this, he had a semi-new procedure done. Electrodes were inserted into his leg, which gave it a small shock that made the foot lift. He could control it from a hand box that fit in his pocket. I was so impressed. I was beginning to understand just how differently everyone experiences MS, and yet we are the same.

When the compression ended, the oxygen started coming through the masks. Steve showed me how to put the mask on and the proper way to breathe through it. I breathed in and out. The breathing was a bit noisy. Steve picked up a book and started reading. I picked up some magazines I had brought in.

My mind quickly wandered off into surreal thought, as usual. I started to think about this scenario. We looked like two old ladies from the 1960s, sitting under hairdryers at a local salon. Instead of having the hairdryers on our heads, they were on our faces. But no, we were actually two strangers with an incurable disease, sitting in a pod together, breathing deeply into masks, while being surrounded by painted pictures of fish. I tried not to laugh. It was curious indeed, yet oddly comforting.

The oxygen infiltration lasted for an hour. After that, the tank started to decompress. The man outside gave a little shout that it was ending, and Steve nodded to me to take off my mask. The decompression took another fifteen minutes, so Steve and I had another chance to chat. We talked a lot about MS, of course. He had very good advice, which I use to this day.

He said, 'With this disease, if you give it an inch, it will park a truck in it.'

The man outside opened the hatch and we exited with our masks in hand. Steve showed me how to take the mask apart and put it in a basin to get cleaned. I was relieved that they do get cleaned actually, because I wondered about that. I went to the bathroom, partly because I always have to pee every hour, and partly because I wanted to look in the mirror. Had the years melted off my face immediately? I was not really expecting to see an instant difference. I *did* see the imprint of the entire mask on my face! But joking aside, I also noticed that I looked more relaxed than usual. *Hmm*

When I came out, I booked for another appointment. They told me that to really see the effects, or should I say *feel* the effects, you have to go for twenty dives in a one-month period. After that, you can go once a week for maintenance. I could not do this, though. It took an hour and a half getting there, an hour and a half getting back, and an hour and a half for the dive itself. I would have to take off work for a month. That was not an option.

I went home that day feeling peaceful and calm. I told William all about my adventure, and he agreed that I looked more relaxed than usual. That night I had one of the best sleeps in my life! I did not wake up during the night to pee! This for me was a miracle. I had woken up to pee every night for the past I don't know how many years. The whole next day, I felt energised. I was truly (and pleasantly) surprised!

The following week, I went for a second session. This time, there were many different people there. Many of them were in wheelchairs. People had different stages of MS. Looking around and meeting everyone, I felt something new. It was guilt. I felt guilty that I was walking, not to mention walking without assistance. Understand that they gave me no reason to feel this way. They were as nice as could be, but I still felt guilty.

I felt like saying, 'Today is a good day for me. You should have met me when I was part blind and stumbling.' I felt like maybe I should limp.

I noticed just then that Steve was there. It was comforting to see a familiar face. The time came and we did our dive together again. We did the same routine: chatted for fifteen minutes, breathed the oxygen for an hour, and chatted for another fifteen at the end. It was soothing and I felt relaxed again.

I walked out without signing up for another session. I liked the actual diving very much, not to mention the after-effects, but I could not shake the guilty feeling. I felt like people in wheelchairs or walking with sticks would not want to see someone with the same disease walking without assistance. I thought I would make them feel bad. I was not sure if I would ever go back.

⅋

For the rest of March I was feeling pretty good. I was happy with my decision to stay in London, even though in the back of my mind I was nervous about the possible risk I was taking with my health. I could not stop thinking about the beta interferons and how I was going to get on them. My mind was put to ease, though, when I received a letter from St. George's Hospital that said I had an appointment to discuss the disease-modifying drugs with a doctor for the 5th of May. That would be five months from my diagnosis, but staying in London was the choice I had made.

My life seemed to be getting back to normal, though. I was working during the day and having fun doing it. The friendliest and coolest celebrities, like Tracy Emin and Paul Weller, were coming in. Sales were going well; the collection was beautiful. I was rehearsing my music at night, and the rehearsals were getting better and better. I was feeling like, *Yes, I can do this! I made the right decision and everything is going to be fine. I am going to beat this!*

Wonderland Again

&

On the 3rd of April, I went to bed feeling fine, except for a minor sore throat that was starting. I gargled with salt water beforehand, which seemed to take it away. I got in bed extra early so that I could wake up fresh and free of a sore throat.

Instead, I woke up in Wonderland again.

The alarm clock went off at the usual time. I opened my eyes and when I looked over to shut it off, there were two clocks instead of one. Again! This time, the two clocks were on top of each other. In my previous episodes, everything was side by side, so up and down was something new.

I immediately realised that I also had a dull pain in the back of my eyes when I turned them.

Shit, I thought. *I don't have time for this. It cannot be happening!* I tried to focus on the clock and make it into one. I could almost do it. I got very close. I got up from the bed en route to the toilet and the room spun all around. Down was sideways and up was sideways. I went tumbling into my closet. Lucky for me, the closet door was open. Also lucky was that my fall was superbly softened by Dolce & Gabbana. Thanks guys!

I picked myself up and stumbled towards the toilet. I smashed into the bedroom doorjamb and then flew into the wall in my hallway. I got to the toilet, sat down, and closed my eyes.

I thought, maybe after I peed I would open my eyes and it would all be back to normal. That thought made no sense, but nothing did at that moment anyway.

No such luck. When I opened my eyes, I still could not focus on anything. There were two sinks on top of each other, two mirrors, two towel racks. You get the idea. I also realised that there were blind spots in my vision as well. One side of my vision had a whole area of darkness.

I burst out crying. I was alone in the house, since William had already gone to work. I started shouting out loud, 'No, no, no! Why is this happening to me?' Then I began an assault of blaring screams at God.

'What the fuck do you want from me? Do you want me to learn something from all this suffering! All I've learnt is that suffering sucks!'

I was slumped over the toilet like a rag doll, weeping uncontrollably. I was in bad shape at that moment. We lived next to an elderly woman, and I can't imagine what she thought from the ruckus.

I got off the toilet and stumbled to the living room. Again, I bounced off of a wall. Not only were things doubled, but also the floor felt and looked like it was on an angle. Walking felt like a cross between climbing and swimming. Climming: a new Olympic sport that I could perhaps win a medal in. I was completely disoriented. I sat on the sofa and closed my eyes again.

William, I wish you were still home, I thought like a lonely howling puppy. It was too early to ring him. He had only been gone for a half-hour, so he would still be on the tube.

The dull pain that had come into my eyes seemed to be getting more intense. My eyes felt like they were held in vice grips. It was fast becoming agonising. While sitting there, staring straight ahead in catatonic misery, I realised that I had yet another visual disturbance as well. I noticed one of the pictures hanging in our living room was floating around by itself. This was the final straw! I could not take it anymore. I was overwhelmed with grief. *Is this how the rest of my life will be? Is this it?* I did not see how I could continue living my life like this. I felt so alone.

I sat on the sofa in a comatose-like state until I got the gumption to get up and ring Simon at work. I dialled the number by the sound of the beeps and mentally knowing where the buttons were.

He picked up quickly.

'It's Marlo. I can't see again,' I told him.

He sounded so sad to hear the crap news. For me, it was beyond disappointing to be in this situation again. I told him I did not know what to do or whom to ring because I really didn't have a doctor. He suggested maybe calling an ambulance, which I considered. I pondered ringing St. George's Hospital, but I hesitated, as my first appointment there was still weeks away. I thought they wouldn't know who I was.

Then I had an idea. I thought I would ring the nurse at the National Neurological Hospital and ask her what I should do. She was used to my ranting from my previous phone calls. That's when a miracle happened. See, they *do* happen!

I rang the number that I had previously called. I did all of this with one eye shut. Because the double vision was up and down, I could not make use of my old glasses, which corrected double vision that's side by side. Closing one eye corrected the problem and allowed me to dial the number.

There was an answering message on, so I left what must have been a pathetic message. 'I am Marlo Parmelee. I am seeing double, I am in pain and I can't walk straight. I don't have a doctor. I am not being treated anywhere. I don't know what to do....' I went on and on.

Twenty minutes later, a nurse rang me back. She told me that I would need to go to the National Neurological Hospital on Tuesday (this was Friday). She explained that they ran what is called a 'relapse clinic' on Tuesdays.

'So, I don't need to go to another hospital?' I asked.

'No,' she said. 'You will be treated at our hospital.'

I couldn't believe what I was hearing. Here I was at one of the lowest points in my life, but now there was hope. I had a place I could go. I had someone to turn to who understood the craziness of this disease. She asked me some questions about what I was going through. Her line of questioning coincided with what I was feeling. I could tell that she knew what she was talking about because her questions were all related to my predicament. She actually understood! She said that another nurse would ring me back to make the appointment.

I hung up not having ever been so relieved in my life. I knew William probably had gotten to work by then, so I rang him.

He could not believe that I was in this condition again. He sounded heartbroken and I am sure he was.

'I'm coming home right now,' he said.

'No way,' I said. 'I don't want you to come home. I am going to sleep anyway. There is nothing that you can do here.'

I didn't think that he should lose a day's pay because of the drama caused by this dumb disease.

Shortly after hanging up with him, the phone rang again. This was the phone call that truly changed everything. It was the woman who would become my MS nurse, Thirusha Lane. She had a kind voice that sounded like she was South African but had lived in England for some time. She told me that I was booked in to the relapse clinic on Tuesday morning.

She also explained to me I needed to rest. Because MS is a disease that inflames the nerves, resting during a relapse can be helpful. I did not realise this until she said it that day. She also asked me if I had any infections, and I said that I had a sore throat. She explained that infections seem to set off MS relapses, and I needed to take care of the sore throat as well. I was amazed by this information.

She then asked me an unusual question, although at the time, I did not think it outlandish because my world was so bizarre anyway. She told me that there was a man filming in the hospital that week for a show called *City Hospital*. This is a daily show on the BBC that visits hospital accident and emergency rooms and films emergencies, with the patient's permission, of course. The show is live on the air. Each show features a pre-taped segment as well. It shows a patient undergoing an operation or a procedure, following the patient for a time period and trying to bring awareness to different medical issues.

So, Thirusha explained that this man would be there taping for the show and asked if I would be interested in being part of it. Lights? Cameras? She did not know me yet.

'Sure,' I said. 'I would be happy to do it.'

Oh dear, I thought, *where's my red lipstick and my bronzer?* Have you ever heard of Touche Éclat by Yves Saint Laurent? It is a light-reflecting make-up product that can make the dead look alive, and I was planning on slapping a whole tube on my face. I swear, if I were on my deathbed and I were offered a chance to be on television, I would gloss myself up even then.

Thirusha explained that it might not even happen, especially if he had enough material with another patient. My thought was, *At this point, I don't really care what happens. My life is already a nonstop roller coaster ride, so what difference does it make? My life is already so weird.*

I spent the rest of the day lying down on the sofa. I got up intermittently for toilet breaks and tea. Each time I got up, my navigational skills were improving. I was able to walk much better just by getting used to the dizziness and double vision. I understood that everything to the left of me was floating in an anticlockwise motion, so I stopped looking to the left. I also remembered some tactics that I had used the previous time, like closing one eye and keeping my hand out in front of me. Once again, this was survival and like the song says, 'I will survive.' Sing it, Gloria Gaynor.

Against my wishes, or should I say my *orders*, William came home early that day. I was never so glad to see the two of him. The two Williams took care of me for the rest of the weekend.

Lights! Camera! Hospital!

∽

The following Tuesday morning, William escorted me to the hospital. I leaned on him the whole way. I could not walk a straight line and I was in a lot of pain. My eyes hurt so badly, worse than the days before. 'I feel like nails are being drilled into the backs of my eyes,' I kept telling William.

'I'm so sorry, little Marlo.' He wrapped his arms tighter around me. 'You will be taken care of soon. They will make you feel better.'

We arrived at the hospital and sat in the same waiting room as when I saw Dr. Palmer. I didn't realise the first time how nice the waiting room was there. It was very modern and calm. The room was full.

'Does everyone here have MS?' I asked William.

'I don't know,' he answered. 'Probably.'

Thirusha, the nurse I had spoken to on the phone, came out to the waiting room to meet us. I liked her even more in person. She was petite and pretty. Her kind voice was accompanied by a warm smile. She sat with us and asked me a few questions about my eyes. She asked me about the severity of the pain and the double vision. Then she told me that I would meet Matt, the guy from the BBC show, before I went into the doctor's office.

She took William and me over to another waiting area where Matt was sitting with his huge TV camera. She introduced us and he gave us a rundown of what *City Hospital* was about.

'I'll be filming you while you're talking to the doctor, if you are OK with that.'

'OK,' I agreed.

'I'll film the examination as well, if you're comfortable with that.'

'Sure,' I said. 'Film whatever you want.'

'I know it's not easy, because you are not actors, but try to act natural in front of the camera. Try to act like it's not there,' he said.

William looked at me, trying not to laugh. *Not actors?* I thought. *I should have worn my Norma Desmond turban. He doesn't realise who he is talking to!*

William squeezed my hand. He knew along what lines I was thinking.

Matt continued, not noticing my little grin. 'I might also interview William, if there's time. Would you be OK with that?' he asked him.

Budding thespian number two will love that, I thought.

'Sure, that's fine,' William, answered.

Matt went on to tell us that what he recorded may or may not air. Sometimes they record things but can't use them. William and I signed a consent form and continued waiting for the doctor.

Matt used the time waiting as an opportunity to ask us some questions about ourselves. He started asking us about our American accents. We began chatting about when we came to England and why. I told him about my music, and he was becoming more and more interested. I was delighted chatting away, because it took my mind off of the pain in my eyes. It also took my mind off of something that was in the back of my mind. I had a sinking feeling that my life was changing in a flash. I was now someone who would probably need periodic hospital treatments for the rest of my life. Again, I had that feeling of the *old Marlo* dying. She was dying, and I was not able to let her go. Not yet.

The doctor finally called us in. Matt followed William and me with the TV camera. Neither William nor I had any trouble acting natural in front of the camera. We pretended it was not there.

The doctor was one whom I had not met before: a young man, blue eyes, very cute. He had a lovely manner too. He started the visit by asking me questions about my symptoms. I had written all my symptoms down as usual, so I took out my papers whilst I answered his questions. I had also drawn a picture of how I saw the world, so I took that out. The drawing looked like the artist was probably on acid, but *I* was the artist, on MS.

William mildly freaked out when he saw it. I could feel him tense up in the seat next to me. I had forgotten to show him my drawing before the doctor visit. He later said that he did not know how anyone could function seeing the world like that. I admit watching objects floating in circles while I am climbing the uphill road that is my living room floor can be quite disconcerting.

After 'the viewing' of my disturbed drawing and some more questions, the doctor began the physical part of the examination. He asked me to walk a straight line, placing one foot in front of the other heel to toe. This was a bit difficult for me. I performed that test with the ease of a slightly intoxicated driver being pulled over by a police officer. I wobbled over to a seat, where the doctor performed several other neurological tests on me.

These types of tests were quickly becoming standard to me. There is one where you touch your finger to your nose and then to the doctor's finger. You continue this back and forth. He also took a piece of cotton wool and touched my face with it, my hands, and so on. He did the same with a sharp object. From these tests, I realised that I had less feeling on one side of my face.

I also had a new symptom. I could not see the colour red properly. Bright reds looked dark red and slightly brown. I hadn't realised it until the exam when the doctor showed me a red object and asked me to describe the colour. This was happening because I had *optic neuritis*, a swelling of the optic nerve that runs behind the eyeball.

'On a scale of one to ten, how bad would you say the pain in your eyes is?' the doctor asked.

'I feel like the back of my eyeballs are being scraped with a potato peeler,' I explained, trying to convey how excruciating it was. 'I would give it a ten.'

It sounds disgusting, but that is exactly what it felt like. The pain was intense and dull. If I moved my eyes sideways, it worsened. It was terrible and it was inescapable.

He looked at my eyes with a small light. I had to follow the light with my eyes. One eye was turning slightly slower than the other. He commented that he could see it kind of sticking. I could feel it pulling. It felt disgusting when I had to turn my eyes slowly for him. The pain mixed with the pulling feeling made me feel nauseous.

I then had to lie down on the exam table while he tested my reflexes and sensitivity on my legs, abdomen, and feet. My infamous left toe was numb again. I started to think how the toe has nine lives because it keeps dying and coming back to life again. He asked me to do other things like run one foot along the other leg. I was not sure if I was passing these tests. I was feeling awkward and felt my movements were not smooth. I was seeing that I had less feeling in general on my left side. My left abdomen did not have a reflex!

After the thorough exam, the doctor confirmed that this was another relapse. He said that the duration of the relapse might be shortened if I took a course of intravenous steroids. He said this could take down the swelling in the nerves quicker than without it and hence speed up the recovery from this episode. I noticed that he was careful to not promise anything, as steroids are actually not *guaranteed* to work. He said if I agreed to take the steroids, then I would need to come back to the hospital for the next three days. They would give me the steroids on an outpatient basis for about an hour and a half a day. It sounded like a great idea to me. All I could think about was getting rid of the intense eye pain as soon as possible.

The next day, William and I made the exact same trip again. We took the bus to the tube while I held on to him for balance. Travelling with him was an indescribable comfort. He was and is my greatest support and always makes me laugh in the midst of the most terrible situations.

When we arrived this time, we had to go to a different part of the hospital. We had only ever been in the outpatient wing. Where we were on this day was a ward where MSers are inpatients. We walked past several beds to where my treatment room was. The room was small and had four big comfy-looking chairs with tables next to them. There was a TV for patient distraction.

We were greeted by Thirusha and introduced to another patient, Terry, who was attached to an IV drip. He was a very nice man in his late thirties. I felt comforted to see another patient getting treatment, although I was sorry that someone else was having a relapse as well.

We sat down and Thirusha explained to William and me exactly what was going to happen and what she hoped the benefits would be. She took her time with us and answered all of our questions. She got me a pillow and blanket and made me as comfortable and as cosy as possible. She then set up an IV bag filled with 1,000 mg of Methylprednisolone, the steroid I was getting.

At this point, Matt arrived with the TV camera. He was just in time to film the insertion. Thirusha inserted the IV into the vein in my arm. She was very good at this. Her method was pretty quick and painless. I told her that my friends at work asked me if I was going to be like 'the Bionic Woman,' after the steroids. They did not realise that the steroids I was receiving were not the same steroids that some athletes take to pump up. Those are metabolic steroids. These were corticoid steroids, which are used to shrink inflammation. We giggled about the confusion.

When the liquid started going into my vein, I felt a slight burn, which Thirusha had warned me could happen. It felt like a hot liquid, but it did not hurt. She also told me that many people get a metallic taste in their mouth. For me, the taste was mild.

We sat there chatting with Thirusha, Matt, and Terry. He and I compared our relapses and talked about the many 'joys' of having MS. His relapse caused one of his arms to spasm, so it was shaking without his control. Because of this, he only had one arm to use for three days of IV therapy. Thirusha had put his IV catheter in his hand, so that he could keep it in for the whole three days. This is a normal procedure that a patient can opt for. I opted for a new insertion into my arm each time. To me, going home with a catheter in me was too gross a thought, even if it was wrapped up in bandages.

Thinking back on this particular experience, I am amazed at the human spirit. Here we all were in this emotionally taxing situation, and yet we coped with it very well. Terry and I were chatting naturally as if we were somewhere else. We just as easily could have been sitting in a room at university waiting for our class to begin. The reality that we were sitting in a hospital room sucking steroids through our veins seemed to vanish. The IVs just disappeared for a while.

I am sure it was not easy for William to watch his wife get hooked up to a drip. It had to be traumatising to some extent, but he handled it with humour, his usual defence. At some points, we would just look at each other and giggle. We didn't need a joke to aid us; we just had to look at each other.

We were all fixated on Terry when he finished his bag of medication. We watched Thirusha detach him from it and bandage him up. When Terry left, Matt began asking William and me questions about how the disease was affecting our lives. We explained that it had only been months since my diagnosis but that we were both very positive about my prognosis.

I felt comforted by the fact that I had a place to go if I relapsed. I also felt comforted by the fact that there was a medication that could speed up the recovery of the relapse. I felt like I was finally being taken care of. Even more encouraging, was that I was suddenly in the *best* of care.

Later that day, I noticed that my eye pain started to lessen. *Am I imagining this?* I thought. I was feeling very good. I was in fact, feeling a little hyperactive. My heart started racing and I began coming up with all kinds of creative ideas. I turned my hyper energies to the computer. With one eye shut, I spent the rest of the day building a new website for Marlo Donato, www.marlodonato.com.

'You should be resting,' William insisted.

'I can't,' I told him. 'I feel jumpy!'

I sat in front of the computer for so many hours, I lost track of time. When I finally stood up, a pain jolted through my back and legs like spears. I suddenly realised that my body was as stiff as a board.

'William, can you come here?' I called out, as I walked hunched over.

'Oh my God,' he said, trying to help me walk to the sofa.

'What the hell is happening to me?' I asked.

William rang Thirusha immediately. She told him that sometimes, although rarely, some patients can have this type of reaction to the steroids. She said I would be given prescription muscle relaxers on top of the steroids the next day. For now, I would need to take over-the-counter drugs.

The next day, Thirusha gave me the muscle relaxers. The rest of the treatment went almost exactly the same as the first day. William, Matt, Thirusha, Terry, and I all sat in the little room chatting, while Terry and I got the drip. In some strange way, I enjoyed it. Sitting with all of them was comforting. Thirusha was taking care of me. William was entertaining me. Terry was in the same boat as me, and Matt was filming me. It was all a comfort.

I got up early on the third day of treatment. I was feeling very good by then, almost high, and I was looking forward to the treatment that day. The pain in my eyes was lessened so much, plus I could move them more easily. My balance was a million times better. I was coming back to the 'real me' at record speed.

The treatment went the same again. All was well. I was a little sad to say goodbye to Terry, when his drip finished and he was bandaged for the last time. We wished each other well and hoped that we would never see each other under these circumstances again. After twenty minutes, my drip also finished and I too was bandaged for the last time.

Before I left, Thirusha told me about a trial they were conducting at the hospital. It was a study for a new version of the beta interferon, Rebif. She gave me some literature about it and told me just to look it over and see if the trial was something I would be interested in taking part in. She explained that unlike in many trials, no one would be on a placebo. Everyone would be on the actual drug. That was because this was the final phase of testing. The drug would probably soon be approved for the masses, or the lucky masses, as it were.

She also told me that the doctor in charge of the study had an incredibly good reputation.

I took the information she gave but thought I would probably not do it. My dad had been on a trial drug for diabetes several years before, and the drug proved to be highly dangerous. That was enough to turn me off drug trials. I walked out thinking, *No thanks!*

Matt filmed William and me leaving the hospital. We left feeling exuberant. I felt so much better after the steroids. Matt asked me on camera how I felt.

'I feel like a person again,' I told him.

We had agreed the day before that if I felt well enough, Matt could come to our flat to film me in my own surroundings. I was feeling wonderful, so we took a taxi from the hospital back to our flat. Matt sat in the front seat and filmed me sitting in the back seat. Again, it was easy to pretend the camera was not there. I just looked out the window and went into my own MS bubble.

He filmed me going into my building, walking up the steps, and entering the living room. He then set his equipment up for a full interview. He instructed me to answer questions with the question in it. For example, if he said, 'What were your first symptoms?' I would say, 'My first symptoms were blah, blah, blah.' Even being in a relapse, I enjoyed being filmed and chatting away.

I answered all the questions and talked about how MS has affected my life. The main idea that I wanted to get across was that getting this disease is not the end of your life. If one person learned something about MS, then appearing on the show would be worth it.

After the interview, Matt filmed me performing daily tasks like making tea and putting on my eye make-up. When I am in a relapse, the eyeliner is a little trickier than usual; the mascara is an extreme sport. I have to put my nose almost against the mirror, shut one eye, and voilà! *Beautiful Marlo in Wonderland!* Who says an awkward bitch can't look good?

He also wanted to film me playing a few of my songs. I happily obliged. I warmed up with one song I wrote called 'Stranger'. I wrote this one the previous summer, before I knew I had MS. I was walking around aimlessly in Pimlico one day, feeling awkward and not knowing why. The first words of the song are 'I'm so numb; I can't feel but tingling in my fingertips.' I meant this literally.

I told Matt not to use that song, because I did not like how I was singing it that day. The high notes were a bit of a stretch considering what I had been through that week. So, I started to sing another one of mine called 'Time Won't Wait'. I was fairly pleased with how I sang that, even though I was starting to get tired.

Matt thanked me for everything and promised that he would let me know when the show would air. When he left, I looked at myself in the mirror and realised that I had bad hair!

Oh no, I thought. *I hope to God that my hair did not look like this when he was filming.* It *did* look like that, as I found out later. And they *did* use 'Stranger'. Damn it.

Charlie's MS Angels

୭

A few days passed and my condition improved tremendously. I was thoroughly impressed by the National Neurological Hospital. I was back at work and functioning semi-normally with only slight wobbling. On this one particular day, actress Katie Holmes came into the shop. She had a fairly large entourage with her, which included bodyguards.

'Is Tom Cruise with her?' a colleague asked. The two celebrities had just broken the news that they were dating.

'I don't think so,' I answered.

'She is very pretty in person,' she commented.

'Yes,' I agreed. 'And ladylike. Well, I am not in a star-struck mood, so I'm off to lunch,' I said. 'However, if Tom Cruise *does* arrive, ring me on my mobile.'

I went to the front door to look at the weather, in case I needed a heavier jacket. The number of paparazzi waiting to see Katie Holmes was enormous. We had plenty of paparazzi many times before, but this was probably the biggest crowd we had in a long time.

'Oh dear,' I said to Colin, looking at the long lenses pointing in at us. They looked like a firing squad.

'What's wrong, Madam? Was Tom Cruise not upstairs?'

'Look at all those photographers,' I said, ignoring his rhetorical question. 'Like hungry wolves. I can't go to lunch until she's gone.'

'Why?' he asked. 'You don't want to give autographs today? Go out. You can practise what it's like. If they don't photograph you, you can say, *Don't you know who I am?*

We both started laughing.

'How dare you!' I said, followed by my well-known precise imitation of Faye Dunaway as Joan Crawford in the film *Mommy Dearest*. 'Christina! Damn it!'

Colin was cracking up laughing now.

'This is serious,' I said. 'I can't get through them. I can't manoeuvre it. What if she comes out at the same time, and in all the magazines, you see me falling behind her? Or you see her looking glamorous and me with a crossed eye behind her?

'Please, darling.' he said, bringing me back down to earth. 'They'll crop you out.'

By the time I got my coat on, Katie was on to the next destination, and so were the paparazzi.

At lunch, I picked up the packet that Thirusha had given me regarding the trial they were conducting at the hospital. I read it over and over. It seemed like it wasn't as much of an experiment as I had thought.

The drug was a version of one that was already on the market and being used worldwide. The difference with this version was that it did not contain an animal-derived protein, or at least that was what I thought I read. *Hmm,* I thought. *It's like the vegetarian version.*

My curiosity was growing. In the back of my mind, I kept thinking about my dad and the trial he had been on. But I decided that I should ring the number on the documents and ask some questions.

I spoke to a lovely nurse called Sara. She explained to me that the trial was called a 'Phase three' trial. This meant that it was in its final stage. There was no placebo in this trial, as Thirusha had mentioned. Everyone who participated in this trial would be on the drug. They already knew that the drug was effective, and this was the final test to see if people develop antibodies to it.

She explained to me that developing antibodies just meant that you could become immune to the drug. Sara told me that the trial would last for two years and that if I was a participant, I would be examined and/or blood tested every three months, as opposed to every six months to a year for regular MS patients.

It seemed very interesting. Sara told me that there were only a few spots left, so if I wanted to be a part of it, I had to say so quickly. I would then need to be assessed by the doctor and approved to be on the drug. Impulsively, I made an appointment to be assessed in two days' time.

At the visit for the assessment, I met Sara, the nurse I was talking to on the phone. The only word to describe her was *cool*. She had long, dark hair with one streak of silver grey in the front. Her pretty face was much too young for this much grey, but it suited her. She was also dressed head to toe in my favourite shade: black. She had a big, welcoming smile.

'You're the television star,' she said, referring to the episode of *City Hospital.*

'That's me,' I said, laughing.

Sara brought me into the office to meet the neurologist in charge of the trial, Dr. Gavin Giovannoni (who is now *Professor* Gavin Giovannoni). He was handsome, maybe in his late thirties, or early forties, with a South African accent. I could tell immediately that he was one of those doctors who became a doctor for the right reason: to help people. He came across as a serious and intelligent person. I could see why he was well respected.

He began to give me one of the most thorough neurological exams that I had ever had. He examined me from my head to my toes. He had a kind nature and a gentle way during the exam. He then sat down and discussed the drug and how I could possibly benefit from being on it. I already knew that I wanted to be on one of the interferons, but I wanted to be cautious and just listen to what he had to say.

'I think that you need to be on one of these drugs, whether it is this one or another,' he said. 'If we look at your rate of relapses, your prognosis is not good.'

What? I thought. *My what is not what?* I wanted to vomit. I had never heard a doctor say anything like this to me. I have never had anything that was more than, 'Not to worry, you're fine.' *How the hell did this become my life?* I pondered. *How did I turn into someone with a bad prognosis?*

'But,' he continued, 'you recover well. Your recovery has been 100 per cent and that is what's on your side.'

At least he does not bullshit around, I thought. I appreciated that he was candid. I realised that he was not being dismal; in fact, he seemed hopeful for me. I appreciated that too.

I took out a list that I had written of about twelve questions. He was happy to answer every single one of them, without rushing me, like many doctors do. I also gave him a diagram that I had skilfully created on the computer of my relapses to date. It was all in colour. I indicated the one month out of the past twelve that I actually felt good with a big yellow smiling sun. I think he and Sara got a kick out of it but also appreciated that I had done a lot of research and took my situation very seriously.

I knew that the trial was the right one for me. Thirusha, the nurse who told me about the trial, was also working on the team. I wanted to be on this drug. I wanted Dr. Giovannoni to be my doctor and I wanted Sara and Thirusha to be my nurses. I signed the consent form and agreed to come back for my first injection on the 17th of May.

Meanwhile, I still had the appointment to see the doctor at St. George's Hospital. I decided to keep it, just to hear what he had to say, since I had waited this long; I might as well meet him too.

William came with me to meet him. We were looking forward to the appointment, as we had read an interesting book that this doctor wrote about MS.

The first thing I said to the doctor was, 'I read your book.'

'That makes two of us,' he replied, dryly.

We found him to be hilarious, as we both love dry humour. I think he had no idea how comical he was. William and I liked him.

He told me that he thought I should be on one of the interferons. I told him that I had the opportunity to be part of this Rebif trial at the other hospital.

'If I were you, I would do it,' he said. He asked what I had to think about. The trial drug was what he called 'Super Rebif'. Well, that was all William and I needed to hear. I would go ahead with my trial at the other hospital. Things were finally moving.

∞

The 17th of May, 2005 was a brisk, sunny day: a perfect day to learn how to inject your own ass with a syringe. My appointment with the MS nurse was at 10 a.m. in the National Neurological Hospital. William and I arrived early.

In the waiting room, there was a very pretty blonde woman, about my age, and her boyfriend. She looked like she could be the actress Scarlett Johansson's sister, maybe even her prettier sister, if that's possible. She seemed to be waiting for the same thing I was, since she was holding an appointment card.

I wasn't convinced, though. She certainly didn't look like she had anything wrong. She looked like she was in perfect physical shape, sitting there, casually chatting with her boyfriend. As I glanced over her, I noticed that she was a true fashionista. She was wearing a beautiful skirt and even more beautiful high-heel shoes.

Well if she has MS, I thought, *she is one fashionable MSer. A girl after my own heart, in fact.*

Maybe her boyfriend has MS, I thought. *No, he looks fine too. They could be waiting for someone to lend support to.*

After a few minutes, another woman came in to the waiting room. She was also pretty, and maybe a couple of years older than us. She looked like she had just gotten off a bicycle, with her little helmet and backpack in hand. *Is she here for the same reason?* I wondered. *She's obviously very fit. Can she have MS?*

William was holding my hand and squeezing it intermittently. He would then smile at me and wink. Once again, he was my support: my buddy, my parent, my husband, all in one.

The nurse came in to the waiting room and looked at all of us. It was Sara, the same nurse I had been speaking with for the past few days.

'Hi everyone,' she said. 'Why don't you all follow me down the hall? Your partners should come as well.'

We all gave a sympathetic glance to one another. Our inner questions were answered. *Yes, we all have multiple sclerosis and we are all here to learn how to inject our own ass.*

We followed her down the hall and filed into an examination room. There were chairs for all of us. I don't think any of us sat back in our chairs, as we were all a bit nervous. William looked like he was already forming questions in his head.

Sara began by introducing us all to each other, as we gave shy hellos. She explained to us that she was going to give us a group instruction first, and that afterwards, we would come in individually and give ourselves the first injection with her supervision. We all nodded approvingly. She also explained that she would be talking more about the drug itself and that she would answer any questions that 'you or your partners might have.'

'Let's begin,' Sara said. 'Now I am going to show you how to inject,' while she proceeded to take out an ambiguous beige object from her desk. It was a square that was about the size of a hand. It looked like it was made out of shiny rubber.

'This is fake skin,' she said, smiling. 'It might look strange, but pretend that it is your leg or stomach. Feel it.' She passed it around and everyone felt its flesh-like texture. We all giggled.

This is when I started to have an out-of-body moment. *OK,* I thought. *I am sitting in a room with six other people. Three of us have an incurable brain disease. We are all sitting around a desk, focused on a slab of fake skin. We will now watch the nurse inject the fake skin and pretend it is our leg or stomach. A little later, we will take a needle and inject it into our real leg or stomach. It will be the first injection of maybe the rest of our lives. OK, Marlo. You can handle this. William is next to you and you are fine. Let's do it!*

I looked around at the two other women. I felt a comfort that not only were we all in the same boat, but they both seemed to have a similar attitude to me—an attitude of 'OK, let's get on with it.' Neither of them seemed sad or mopey in any way. They did not seem that scared either.

Sara's voice interrupted my inner dialogue.

'The first thing to do is to always wash your hands. Just use soap and water. Now watch me carefully.'

We were intently focused on her desk. Next to the fake skin was a green box with what looked like a giant pen in it. It was in fact, a type of 'injector pen' called the *Rebiject*, made by the same company that manufactures the drug itself. The pen came in two parts.

'First you take this part and hold it upright.' She was holding the fatter of the two ends. 'With your finger, push down the trigger to ready the mechanism.' She pushed down the inner part, which was on a spring.

'Next take out your pre-filled syringe.' Our medication was in pre-filled syringes, so we never had to worry about measuring or mixing anything. The syringes were made of glass and had a pink sticker indicating that it was a test drug. The liquid inside was colourless.

'Now, what you do is put the entire syringe, with the safety cap on, into the front part of the injector pen.' She placed the syringe into the skinnier part of the pen. 'But in the first months, you are all going to slowly wean onto the drug. You will start with a quarter dose, and then go up to a half dose, leading up to a full dose. This is called titration.'

Again, she explained that we did not have to measure anything. There was a small clip that we had to put on the syringe that would only allow a certain dosage to shoot out of it. They were colour coded too: white clips for the quarter dose and green ones for the half. It looked pretty easy so far. After she placed the syringe into the skinnier half of the pen, she took the other half and screwed it together. When it was together, it was about the size of a carrot.

How will she get the safety cap off of the syringe? I wondered.

'On the tip of the pen, there is a small grey cap, you see?' She showed us the attached cap. 'When you pull it off, the safety cap on the needle will automatically come off and you are ready to inject.'

Impressive, I thought. *They have made this as easy as possible.*

'Next you hold your skin between your thumb and pointer finger, pulling it away from the muscle, like this.' She demonstrated on the fake skin slab. 'Hold the pen at a ninety-degree angle and press the release button. The needle will go into your skin. Wait a few seconds for all the medication to go in. You should then gently rub your skin to help the medication spread.' The button was at the top of the pen. When she did it on the fake skin, the needle seemed to go in at an amazing speed.

I started to think, *Was there real medication in that one she just used? It couldn't possibly be. This would be an expensive demonstration.*

'I'm going to do it again,' she said. 'By the way, these syringes that I am using today are filled with saline, not medication. They are just for demonstration.' Question answered.

She did the procedure again and instructed us to put the empty syringes into a 'sharps bin' afterwards. She said we would each be given little bins to take home. 'Now it is your turn.'

I imagined the three of us as *Charlie's Angels* (the original show) with our trigger fingers at the ready. Nurse Sara was *Bosley,* of course. I wanted to say something to them like 'Ladies, let's inject.' I refrained.

One at a time, we got closer to her desk and tried out the procedure. We each successfully injected the piece of rubber with the saline. We looked at each other approvingly. We each seemed ready to try the real thing on ourselves.

Cecile, the woman with the bicycle helmet, was asked to stay in Sara's office to try her first real injection. The rest of us shuffled off into the waiting room.

'I feel very lucky to be part of this study,' Kate (Scarlett Johansson's would-be sister) said to us. She told us how she found out she had MS. There were huge similarities to my story and huge differences as well.

I liked Kate's attitude. It was similar to mine. We chatted about when and where we were diagnosed, and how we felt. I was delighted to meet her. For the first time, I felt like I met someone who has MS and is just like me. She was not going to let it stop her life in any way. She also had a partner who was supportive, like William.

My turn came to try the injection on myself. I wanted to be perfect, just for the sake of being a good student. I went through all the steps, as William watched and Sara coached. I put the filled injector pen up against my stomach and *swish!* I did it! I felt almost nothing. There was no pain, almost no sensation at all. *OK, I can do this for the rest of my life,* I thought. *This is nothing.*

Sara gave us a small silver cooler bag to put the medication in. (I later used it for four-packs of Guinness as well.) She gave me cards that I had to fill in every day, if necessary, to record my symptoms, when I injected, and other medications I took. We put the boxes of syringes into the bag and we were off.

'I did it!' I said to William as we walked out of the hospital.

'I am so proud of you,' he said, hugging me.

'What shall we do now?' I asked.

'Let's go get abused by the little Italian man at the sandwich shop.' he answered.

I laughed. 'You took the words right out of my mouth!'

We entered the coffee shop and witnessed the man verbally abuse all the customers as usual. We had our tea and little sun-dried tomato sandwiches. I was now officially on medicine. The medicine that I had waited so long to be on was flowing somewhere inside my body. All was well with the world for now.

Later that night, I began to feel the side effects of the medication. During the visit earlier that day, Sara told us what the possible side effects of the injection could be. 'Flu-like symptoms' such as chills, headache, and body aches were some of the possible ones. For me, that was something of an understatement. I had no idea what I was in for.

Permanent Flu

ം

The next couple of months became a permanent flu. On a Monday, Wednesday, and Friday night, I would do my usual things, such as eating, laughing with William, and Internet surfing. At around 9 p.m., I would take two Nurofen, as a precautionary measure against the pain that Rebif would first bring. At around 10 p.m., I would inject myself, either in my stomach or one of my legs.

Each time I injected, the medication would leave a pink spot the size of a fifty-pence coin. On me, the spot would stay for about three weeks. I was instructed not to inject into a pink spot, so after a month, my search for a spotless area started to become a challenge. I was covered in pink spots! I was like a polka-dotted person! I also broke capillaries in some of my injection areas, so I had bruises as well.

Sometimes when I got out of a hot shower and looked in the mirror, I would gasp. I looked like I had been beaten. The pink spots and bruises were bright and huge!

Shortly after realising how quickly the spots multiplied, I started injecting my ass. I found humour in the fact that I injected my own ass. In fact, to this day, while I am doing it, I laugh every time.

'Look what my life has come to!' I say out loud. 'Injecting my own ass!'

In the beginning, there was almost no pain in the actual injection. (That changed after a couple of years, but not to worry, I am used to it now.) After each injection, there would be a lump under the skin where the protein was hanging out for a while. I massaged this to make the liquid disperse into the skin a little easier. This part was mildly painful, but overall it helped.

All would be well for about an hour. After that, a feeling of being unwell would start to creep into my body, like a camouflaged enemy sneaking in. You know the feeling when everyone at work has the flu, and you decide that you are too strong to get sick? Then you come home from work feeling light headed and sluggish. You are on the verge of getting chills, as your eyes start to burn. Slowly you realise that you are getting it too. You try to fight the malady sweeping over you until you have to give in to the fever, chills, headache, and body aches. Do you know that feeling?

Multiply it by 100 and you'll come close to how I felt. I had pain in so many parts of my body. Even my hair hurt. Every muscle felt like it was stretched on a rack. The tip of my nose hurt, my chin hurt, my teeth hurt. My eyes hurt so badly. My back probably hurt the most.

One night I woke up thinking that my fingers had little brains in them, and each one had a headache. Even my fingernails hurt. Breathing hurt. Thinking hurt. Touching the sheets hurt. I could not find a position to relieve the agony.

Then the chills would come. I would start shaking out of control. If I was asleep before all these symptoms started, then I would wake myself up moaning or shaking or crying. I woke up William every time, either accidentally or on purpose. He would get up and get me more painkillers. I started to live on Nurofen. I would 'top up' on the pills and wait. This lasted for usually three hours, and sometimes I would get to sleep and sometimes not.

I adopted a new way of sleeping standing up. In fact, I thought about installing a hook on my wall so that I could wear a hoodie and hang from it. I would stand with my bum directly on the wall heater. The heat seemed to soothe my back pain. I could start to fall asleep like that. Sometimes I would just lean forward and stretch my upper body to where the bed was. I could lean over and put my head on the bed, propped up on pillows, while my lower body stood at the heater. It was very hard.

Once again, the thought of suicide seemed like a good idea. The contemplation was not one of sadness, but one of escapism.

I thought, *OK, I got this stupid disease, well fuck it then, I am getting off this ride.*

I started to feel isolated as well. The problem is on a Tuesday morning, no one cares that you spent Monday night in this condition. No one can understand what you've been through, and now your physical pain becomes emotional pain as well.

It is my nature to share my experience with others, usually to the point of vulgarity. But how many times can people hear that you had a bad night? This is one reason why people with MS suffer in a sort of silence. It is a chronic disease, but you can't be a chronic complainer about it. Some people believe that we suffer in this life in penance of sins from past lives. If that is true, then I must have been one serious bitch!

ॐ

The summer was turning out to be exhausting. On the 7th of July, I woke up feeling just as tired as usual. William was also not feeling well. We thought about not going to work and spending the day together. Instead, we dragged ourselves out of the bed. William got ready quickly and left to get the tube.

About ten minutes later, he rang me to tell me not to try to take the tube. There were major delays, which happen often, and they were not letting people into our station.

'Thanks for telling me,' I said.

He told me that he was going to get on a bus.

William often rang me from his commute to warn me about areas to avoid. It was helpful to me on many occasions. I continued getting ready for work.

Another ten minutes went by and he rang again. This time he told me that he could not get on any buses. They were all so full, that the drivers were not stopping.

'Come home,' I said. 'You see, we should have stayed in bed.'

He told me that he would probably come home and wait for rush hour to be over.

I started on my way to work. I went immediately to a bus stop where I knew there would be fewer people. There was still a fair crowd waiting, but at least I got on the 137 bus. Traffic seemed to be moving slowly and the bus was stopping at every stop for people. I rang work to tell them that I might be a few minutes late. The person who answered told me not to worry; everyone was running late. There was some kind of problem with the transport system that day. He said that most tubes were shut down.

When the bus got to Sloane Square, I noticed that the tube station there was now open. *Ooh! This is perfect! I* thought. I jumped off the bus and ran into the tube. Now I would be in work in five minutes.

I got onto a Piccadilly line train that was just about to close its doors. The door message sounded, but then the doors stayed open. *Come on,* I thought, hastily. A couple of minutes went by and more and more people were running for the train. It's always anticlimactic when you run and jump on a train, but then the door does not shut behind you. Everyone had that 'Why the hell did I just run and jump?' look on their face.

As I stood there in the train, I started to get a bad feeling. *Something is wrong,* I thought. I panicked and jumped off the train. *I'll let this train go. I'll stand on the platform and wait for the next. This one might get stuck in the tunnel.*

I was off the train for less than a minute when they announced in the station that everyone was being evacuated. We were all used to things like this happening for whatever reason. You know, a package was left unattended and now we have to evacuate, kind of thing. This seemed different, though. Everyone looked too calm. They looked more put out than concerned. My instincts told me that despite the casual pace everyone was evacuating at, something was really wrong.

When I got out of the tube station, I darted for another bus. Now I was on my way to work again. The bus driver had his CB radio on quite loud and seemed to be focused on the intense conversations being broadcast over it. The whole bus could hear what his colleagues were saying. I heard one voice say, 'Just let people on the bus without paying. You have to get as many people away from it as possible!'

We all looked at each other. Everyone started asking, 'What is going on? What do people need to get away from?'

Then someone said, 'London is being bombed by terrorists.'

We're being what by what? I thought. *Oh shit, here we go again.*

During the terrorist attacks on September 11, 2001, I was employed in Manhattan and also trying to get in to work. I hoped that this was not happening in London, but I had a sinking feeling in my stomach.

I rang William immediately. He was home. I told him to stay where he was and turn on the radio. He told me to get off the bus and come back home. I told him that I was almost at my job. I would go in and see what the whole story was.

When I got to work, people were saying that several bombs had gone off throughout London. The story kept changing as to how many and where they went off. We opened the shop but just kind of stood in a circle, ringing people we knew to see if they were all right and to tell them that we were OK. I rang my mom in the States. It was just before 6 a.m. in New York. I knew she usually gets up at 7 a.m., but I did not want her to turn on the television without talking to me first.

She said, 'Is everything all right? You are calling early.'

I started making jokes, so that she would hear that I was fine. Then I said, 'I'm just calling to tell you something that happened here this morning. I don't want you to turn on the news and hear it there. William and I are totally fine, but there have been some bombs set off on the tube this morning.'

'Oh no,' my mom said. She started crying. I knew she was remembering September 11. She was grounded in Ireland at that time, as she had gone over for her brother's funeral. It was hard for her to be there while my sisters and I were at home in New York. Now it was happening again, only I was the one on this side of the pond.

She kept saying, 'I wish I was there with you. I love you. You'll be all right.' We hung up like we might never see each other again.

I felt sick then. The whole situation started to hit me hard. God knows how many people had died at that point. It was devastating. People were scared. It was a volatile situation.

We closed the shop a few minutes later. Simon said that our sister shop in Knightsbridge was staying open if anyone wanted to come over there with him and work. *Fuck that,* I thought. *I have seen this situation before.* I started to think about what happened in Manhattan when the whole city was on lockdown. No one could get in or out.

Bridges are always the most vulnerable spots, so I thought there was a chance that they would close the bridges in and out of central London. This was exactly what had happened in Manhattan on September 11. William and I lived in Clapham Common, south of the river. All I could think about was getting over the Chelsea Bridge, getting home, and holding William.

One girl I worked with, Nancy, lived near me in Clapham. We decided that we should walk home together. Everyone was out on the streets walking, as the buses also stopped running. It was pouring rain also. I stopped in Starbucks to get my comfort coffee, the beloved Caramel Macchiato. I needed fuel for the long walk home.

During the walk, the thought that I had MS did not cross my mind once. I had a goal in my mind. The goal was to get this girl and me over the Chelsea Bridge, and that was it.

The first part of the walk was fine. We passed by many clothing shops, looking in all the windows. We talked about clothing a little, but mostly about what was happening. It was a surreal situation. You would think I would be used to these surreal situations by then, but this was just out of control. As we got down into the heart of Knightsbridge, Nancy started to complain.

'I am getting very tired,' she said.

'We have to keep going,' I told her. 'Don't tell me about tired,' I said under my breath. 'You don't know fucking tired.'

'We are almost at the bridge,' I said out loud, trying to sound positive and peppy.

She started stopping every few feet and looking for taxis.

'All the taxis are full,' I told her. I was starting to wish that I were by myself. She did not respond to my pep talks as well as I myself responded to them.

'Come on,' I said. 'If I can do this, you can do it. Keep walking!'

What I really wanted do was start screaming, 'Get your ass over that bridge, missy! I have a fucking brain disease and you don't see me complaining, do you? Move, soldier!'

I kept these words to myself. Instead, I just kept walking. She would have to catch up. So, we started walking over the bridge. The rain was coming down sideways and the wind was strong over the water. We were soaked, but I did not care. My eye was on one thing and one thing only: the other side of the river.

A few minutes after we got to the other side, Nancy was looking for taxis again. I kept walking until I heard her call my name. She had actually managed to get one! *I'll be damned,* I thought. *I guess I should have had more faith in her.*

I got home and flung my arms around William. 'I love you! I love you!' we said, kissing every inch of each other's wet faces. We cried so much. All of our inner pain and life turmoil was overshadowed by the senseless deaths of all these innocent people. We were sickened by the stupidity and evilness of mankind. MS meant nothing to us at that moment.

Summer

ଊଠ

'What were you thinking wearing that ratty jumper?' Colin asked. He was referring to my appearance on *City Hospital*, which had now aired. I had indeed made a poor fashion choice in one of the segments. I had not seen the show yet, but Colin had taped it for me.

'We cried through the whole thing,' he said.

'Because of the jumper?' I joked.

'You are a strong woman,' he said. 'And to see how William supports you so much.... and when he said *She has MS, but MS doesn't have her!* Oh, darling, we were sobbing our little hearts out.'

'Please stop or *I* will start crying,' I said before changing the subject. 'Did my hair look crappy in the segment where I was playing my songs?'

'It was a little wonky,' he answered, truthfully. 'You could've done with a stylist.'

'Damn it,' I blurted. 'Did they show me singing "Time Won't Wait"?'

'Yes, and also the one where you sing about being a stranger.'

'Damn it! That's the one I asked him *not* to use! Oh well.'

I received many positive responses from friends and family who saw the show. People told me that they learned a lot about multiple sclerosis, and that made me feel good. *It was worth it,* I thought. *Worth the bad hair!*

ဢ

Days later, William and I were in New York for a holiday. When I walked out of JFK airport, the heat hit me like a slap in the face. This was not normal heat. This was over thirty degrees Celsius with 100 per cent humidity. It felt good for about sixty seconds.

Almost immediately, my left leg started to feel heavy and lose feeling. I was so happy to see my sisters waiting for me, but as I approached them, I thought, *OK, what the hell is happening to my leg?* I tried to ignore it. By the time I got to my mom's house, my leg was feeling like someone else's leg. I was losing so much sensation in so short a time. I was like a different person.

I had read earlier that heat can have a negative effect on MS. I thought I would be fine in the heat, since I had felt great in Miami months before. I learned my lesson, though. Mild heat with low humidity is fine for me. Extreme heat, or actually any heat that is coupled with high humidity, is my nemesis.

I was having a great visit with my family, but the leg was constantly on my mind. For the first couple of days, the numbness was from my toes to my knee on the left leg. The numbest part was my toes. The big toe, which was the first part of me to ever go numb, was completely dead. Once again, I was expecting it to turn blue. This was its fourth, fifth, or maybe sixth death! I had lost count.

The heat continued to hold up in New York. I talked with my mom about how I used to live for the sun. The hotter it was the better. At one time, I was a hard-core sun worshipper. I would mix baby oil with iodine to get a deep, dark tan. I thrived in hot weather. That all seemed to be changing now. Again I felt this sense of mourning for the *old Marlo*. The Sun Goddess was officially dying. I was not sure who this new girl would be, but she was destined to be pale for the rest of her life!

After maybe the third day in New York, the numbness actually got significantly worse. It crept higher and higher up my leg. Walking became more difficult.

I had planned to go shopping that day, so I was not going to let it stop me. I took my mom's car keys and walked out the front door. When I turned off of the front steps, I almost fell over into the bushes. It was a sight to behold. I went back in the house and sat down. My mom was upset by what happened. I was actually a bit confused by how quickly I was falling to shit. I remembered that my mom kept my grandfather's old walking stick in a closet somewhere. I, of course, found it and headed back out with the stick to the shops. It did not cross my mind to not go shopping. In fact, I felt like dark forces were challenging me. They were trying to keep me from great sales and new shoes. *Well, screw them*, I thought. *I will not be stopped.*

'Mom,' I called through the car window. 'My mission today is to buy 200-dollar shoes for 40 bucks and this shit is not going to stop me!' With that, I drove off.

By the fifth day, I could barely feel my left buttock. Not to be crass, but I could not feel my left labia majora either. This was a bit alarming. *This had better go away,* I thought, *or it could be a real bad problem! If it spreads elsewhere, things could get even worse for me.*

Can it go into my clitoris? I thought. This thought made me very upset. As usual, I started to laugh out of control. I made jokes to my sisters about it. We were all laughing, and all wondering too.

'I thought MS was bad before today. This disease is really starting to suck.' I told them. 'And *suck* is all I will be doing, if my clitoris is not working.'

Our holiday only lasted for six days, although because of my downward spiral, that was ample time. We had arranged that my mom would fly back with William and me. We would take her to Paris for her seventieth birthday. I was so glad to be going on the plane with her. I used the walking stick in the airport. It was very helpful. As usual, I was concerned about my look. I thought the stick looked cool, surprisingly. I told myself that if someone asked me what had happened to my leg, I would say I had surgery after an injury from some extreme sport. 'You've got to watch those moguls!' I could say. 'My snowboard cracked in half!'

No one asked, and I am sure no one cared.

When the plane took off, I felt a sense of relief and sadness. I was glad to be out of the New York heat. I don't think I could have taken another day. I was sad to leave my sisters again, though. The biggest sadness, however, was that I knew this was the last time I would ever go home in the summer. This thought broke my heart. On Long Island, the summer was always the best time. It was the time I missed the most when I was in England. I always daydreamed about the beach at home. Now I knew that unless a cure for MS is found, I would not go back to those beaches, at least not in the summer. I was now starting to hate what I used to love. A little more of the *old Marlo* died.

ઈ

During the time my mom was in London with me, the National Neurological Hospital was giving seminars for people who were newly diagnosed with MS. William and I attended almost all of them, and now my mom got to go as well. They were informative and gave us the opportunity to meet other people who were newly diagnosed. As I attended these seminars, I observed my mom listening attentively to the information regarding the disease her daughter had. She looked so positive smiling in her chair, but it broke my heart. The realisation that I have a disease sunk in a little more.

In fact, after my mom went back to America, the realisation hit me several more times. One significant time was when a woman rang me from the Red Cross, because I had signed up to donate blood. She told me when the next donation date was, and I agreed to go.

'There is one thing,' I told her. 'I don't know if it matters, but I have been diagnosed with multiple sclerosis. It is not contagious.'

'Will you hold for one moment?' she asked.

She came back a minute later. 'I am very sorry,' she explained. 'But you won't be able to donate blood. I'll update our list.'

'*I* am very sorry,' I told her. 'I wish I didn't have this disease and I could donate.' I started to cry.

'I am so sorry,' she said again.

I hung up in a bit of a daze. I put my head on the table and continued crying. *I am off the list. They don't want my blood because I have a disease.*

'I have a disease,' I said out loud. Another little part of the *old Marlo* died.

₧

After nearly three months of injecting Rebif, my symptoms seemed to subside. It almost happened overnight. I woke up one morning feeling fine, and I later realised that I had injected the night before. *Holy crap! I actually injected the night before and felt fine in the morning!* This was a big deal. I had not felt that good in three months. I felt like I was coming back to the land of the living.

For one week, I felt incredible. I was running around at work in my four-inch heels again. I was coming home and helping William cook and do the dishes; two tasks I had stopped doing.

We were going out to dinner and taking walks in the evening. My eyes were looking bright. I had energy. I did what many women do to mark a new me. I coloured my hair. I looked and felt terrific.

It did not last. A couple of days before my three-month follow-up appointment with the doctor, I started to have a weird feeling in my right eye. I actually convinced myself, yet again, that a piece of dust was in it. I felt so good. The thought of another relapse was not on my mind, or at least not in forefront.

When I looked to the right, I was cocking my whole head, without realising it. There was a pulling feeling in my eyes. When I would turn my eyes, I sometimes heard a sound in my head. It was a wet squeaky door. It was not loud, but it was gross.

I started to notice an odd feeling on my forehead also. I had a ticklish, yet burning, itch. I could not stop scratching my hairline. I thought it was perhaps from the hair dye. When I scratched it, it felt like I was scratching the wrong spot. It is hard to describe. I knew where the itch was, but scratching it did not relieve it. It might have made it worse, actually. When I touched the itchy spot, it did not even feel like my skin. The itch didn't feel like an itch anymore. I felt like the itch would faintly travel to other parts of my face as I was scratching it. It was bizarre. I kept telling people, 'I have this mad, *un-scratchable* itch!' It was driving me crazy. I never assumed that it had anything to do with my MS, so I tried to dismiss it.

While I was outdoors, I seemed to have a more intense itch if the wind was blowing in my hair. It started to feel more painful. It depleted my spirit because the wind in my hair was always one of my favourite feelings. It represents freedom. Now I felt like this freedom was being taken from me. I stopped brushing my hair too, as the brush gliding on my scalp seemed to have the same painful effect as the wind blowing.

While out walking on the street, I was tripping everywhere again. I could not walk a straight line if I tried. The awkward bitch was back. One morning I thought about buying a can of beer to carry with me. I was sure people thought I was recovering poorly from a night of binge drinking. *I might as well carry the evidence with me.*

When I went to the three-month appointment for the Rebif trial, I was having what I thought was a pretty good day. I was feeling fine, except for the weird eye feeling and the scalp pain (yes, that's all). I thought I would simply go there, get checked, and pick up my next three months of medication. I told Thirusha, about my weird eye and scalp feeling. When I am at the doctor's, I never remember all my symptoms. I usually write them down beforehand. I did not this time, because I felt that they were mild and insignificant.

As I started telling her what had been happening, I realised that I was probably having another relapse. I felt like bursting into tears. My heart sank to my stomach. I could feel my face heating up. I felt like a failure. I had let everyone down, including myself. *Everyone will be so disappointed*, I thought. *I* was sorely disappointed.

Thirusha told me that she was making an appointment for me in the relapse clinic. That word started to sound different in my ears. Instead of 'relapse clinic', I heard it as 'You're a pathetic failure clinic'. Maybe it should be called 'Your lousy immune system has fucked you over again clinic'. Better yet, it could be called 'Abigail partied with her fucking friends, and you're in her hangover clinic'. I was filled with grief.

When I left the office, I felt like ditching work. I was walking in a daze. I looked well enough, but here I was walking around London feeling peculiar once again. My head was dancing with thoughts. I thought of William.

'Hi, honey I'm home!'

'How was your day, Marlo?'

'Great! I'm relapsing again, but other than that, everything is just dandy!'

Maybe I could just lie this time, I thought. *Maybe no one needs to know*. I wondered if I avoid telling William. Impossible.

Thirusha had just given me three more months' supply of syringes filled with Rebif. I carried them in the silver cooler bag. *Just the kind of thing you want to be carrying on the tube when the police are looking for suspicious bags,* I thought.

Police were in Green Park tube station with sniffer dogs, all because of the heightened terrorist alerts after the bombings of 7 July. Luckily, I looked innocent enough, except for the slight stumbling.

At one point, I stopped to buy a bowl of porridge. I thought it was bizarre to be walking around with a bowl of porridge in one hand and £4,000 of drugs in the other. I tried to make myself laugh thinking about it, but instead, I started crying.

I arrived at work and made myself a cup of tea. Only one person saw me crying: Dan, the poor guy who always witnessed my kitchen mishaps. He gave me a look of 'Should I stay with you?'

'I'll be all right,' I whispered to him and he left the room. I sat down and gave myself one of my pep talks. *You will pull yourself together. You will pick your heart up off the floor, put on your red lipstick, and get moving.*

It is good to cry when you have to. Since having MS, I am not sure if I cry more or less than I did without MS. It might be less. I feel like I am crying over the same thing sometimes. How many times can you cry over the same subject?

I pondered the thought of how relapsing-remitting MS is like being in a bad relationship. Sometimes everything is great, and life is fantastic. Other times, you are treated like crap and wonder how you ever got there. You cry every time, even though essentially you are crying over the same thing. It will never get better, and your friends keep telling you that you are beating a dead horse. It is a cruel, vicious cycle. Unlike a bad relationship, though, you cannot get away.

I returned to the shop floor and carried on my day as usual. The UK area manager rang and asked how my doctor's appointment went.

I said, 'OK. I am just having a little trouble with my eye again, so I have to go back to the relapse clinic next week.'

There was a long pause on the other end.

'Hello?'

'How can this be?' he asked finally. 'How is this possible? I thought you are on medication now.'

I explained to him that this is what happens in relapsing-remitting MS. One day you can be fine, and the next, you are in a relapse. The medication is *not* a cure. He did not understand and I was getting angry.

'This is too bad,' he said. 'You must be very disappointed.'

'Yes,' I snickered. *What the hell?* I thought. *I must be very disappointed? You don't know what disappointed is!*

Drug Land

&

The next day, I woke up feeling even weirder. My eye was partially paralysed again. Sixth nerve palsy was obviously back.

I tried to find humour, as usual. I pretended to make an announcement at a fictional American supermarket. 'Clean up in aisle six,' I said sounding like an elderly lady with a clothes peg over her nose. 'We've got a nerve spill in aisle six!'

William laughed at my joke, as he performed all the usual eye tests on me to see how bad it was. I followed his finger from side to side. The paralysed eye muscle was not as bad as it was in the past, but the pain was getting there. I felt crappy.

I called in sick that day. Simon seemed disenchanted. His boss, the UK area manager, was also there that day. He still did not understand that beta interferon is not a cure. He was questioning why I would have eye problems again when I was on a medication. I certainly did not have the patience to explain it to him that day. I had tried to explain it to him the previous day and he wasn't getting it.

I rested all day, but stupidly went to work the next day. I was struggling, as the pain was getting worse. The pain was not exactly the same as before. The intense dull ache was back, but this time it was coupled with some stabbing pains, especially in my teeth. I had stabbing pains in my eyes, nose, and jaw, yet my cheeks were a bit numb.

My face was starting to feel like its own entity. I visualised screwdrivers up through my eyelids. The painful itchiness on my scalp now intensified to full-on pain. It was like pins in my head. I took so many painkillers but they were not working. I started to wish that my head could be chopped off temporarily.

Later at work that day, I received a phone call from a friend from New York who was visiting London. He was my old bass player, Dave. I knew that he and his friend were planning a visit to London, but with all the pain and weirdness, I had forgotten. They had landed that morning. William and I had been begging Dave to visit us for over a year, and now here he was! But now I felt like crap! Great!

Dave and his friend were only in town for two days, as they were on a European tour. William and I wanted to see them. Dave asked how I was, so I just lied.

'I'm fabulous!' I said, and I made dinner plans for that night.

Later on, William wondered how I was going to pull this one off. 'Why don't we just tell him that you are not well? Maybe we can just have them over for a drink, so you can rest in the house.'

'No way,' I said. 'We have been asking him to visit us since we first moved here and now here he is. I love Dave and I am not going to crap out on him. He is here to have a good time, and a good time he will have. We are going out and I am not telling him any bad news.'

So we went out to dinner and I pretended that there was nothing wrong with me. I did not want to explain it. I did not want to disappoint Dave, either. He knew I had been doing so well, and I could not let him down.

I struggled for most of the night, pretending that I was not in pain. This was strongly aided by stout, of course. The stout did not take away the pain, but it took away the care that I had pain, and that was good enough for me.

After dinner, we took Dave and his friend on the London Eye. What was interesting about being in the pod at the London Eye was how good it felt. Any time I was in an unusual surrounding, I felt pretty good.

For example, there is a shop in Camden called Cyberdog, where they blast rave music so loud that you have to use sign language to speak to the salespeople. The floor actually shakes with the vibrations. When I am in that shop, I feel normal. The vibrating floor helps me feel centred, like I can walk straight.

The pods of the London Eye had the same effect. They move very slowly. Most people say that they do not feel like they are moving at all. There is, however, a minuscule amount of buoyancy to the pod. Scientifically, I guess there just has to be, right? This small amount of vibration offset my awkwardness. It made me feel good.

I thought about living in the pod. It was big enough to be a small flat. *I could set up a bed and toilet in one of them,* I thought. *I could have a tiny kitchen too. Yes, I could live inside the London Eye, with my bad eye. How ironic.*

Disembarking was sad. I wanted to have another go-round. I wanted to feel normal again, but all good things come to an end. When we were all getting back on the tube and saying farewell, Dave said, 'I am glad to see you doing so well! Lucky you are on that medicine.'

'Yes, Lucky,' I said, and smiled inside. He never knew.

☙

In the days that followed, the pains in my face got weirder and stronger. I went to the relapse clinic, which I was no longer calling the 'failure clinic', and saw Dr. Giovannoni. He performed many tests on me, including rubbing cotton wool on my cheeks, which I did not really feel. My infamous toe with the nine lives was also dead again. The L'Hermitte's sign was also back. You know the one where I put my head down to my chin and feel the zap? Love that one.

'You are having a relapse,' Dr. Giovannoni said. He questioned me about the pain in my face. He wanted to know if I took anything for the pain. I told him that I tried Panadol and Ibuprofen, but they did not seem to work.

'They won't work on this,' he explained. 'They cannot help neuropathic pain. I am going to give you a prescription.'

He explained to me that he was prescribing a drug called Neurontin. It is a drug that is sometimes given to epileptic patients. In fact, it is technically an anticonvulsant. But it is used to relieve neuropathic pain as well. It sounded good. Truthfully, a gun would have sounded just as good.

When I picked up the medicine at the hospital pharmacy, I noticed that the diagnosis on the prescription read more than 'MS relapse.' It also read, 'trigeminal neuralgia.' I remembered seeing this word on an MS website, which talked about excruciating facial pain. Apparently, trigeminal neuralgia is also known as 'the suicide disease'.

I had to wean onto the drugs, which I started immediately. The first day, I felt good. I still felt pain, but I also felt slightly high. By the fourth day, when I was on the full dose, I wanted to tell everyone that I loved him or her. I could not stop smiling. I felt so sleepily happy. I thought I was on a cloud or a big billowy bed, but alas, I was actually at work, trying to conduct myself accordingly.

Because of the highness factor, working on this drug was a bit tricky. Days off were OK, though. One day, William took me to the Royal Botanic Gardens at Kew (Kew Gardens). This is one of the most beautiful botanical gardens in Great Britain. We could not believe how big it was as we walked through it. It even has redwood trees from California!

I could not stop smiling. There were so many colours and species to take in and I was so damn high. I was a bit drowsy though. Luckily, there are benches aplenty at Kew Gardens. I think I rested on all of them.

As we walked along, I would focus on a tree or a flower and say to William, 'Let's sit on this bench and admire nature.'

At one point, we went into the giant greenhouse there. It was magnificent. It had an exhibit of glass art that month. Handmade glass flowers and ferns were mixed in with the real ones. It was beautiful, but I started to feel weird looking at them. I began thinking that the real flowers should not be disturbed by the glass ones. I started to imagine the real flowers getting angry at the glass ones and wanting the glass ones to leave.

'This is not natural,' I told William, angrily. He started laughing.

'No,' I said. 'This is not funny. They are very saddened.'

'Who's saddened?' he asked. 'The flowers?'

'Yes, the flowers!' I said sternly. I was disgusted.

Near the exit of the greenhouse, there was a guest comments book. William wrote something like 'Very beautiful. Thanks!' I wanted to write something like that, but on this drug, my mind had fewer filters. I wrote something a little rude about the unnaturalness of glass posing as plants. I also wrote how the real flowers were not happy because of it.

'What did you write?' William asked, noticing I took a little extra time.

I started laughing like a stoned person. I was laughing slowly. I would let out one 'ha' and then pause a moment. After the pause, I would let out another 'ha.'

'What are you doing?' he asked. 'You are laughing like a nut. What did you write?'

When I told him, he did not believe me at first.

'I hope you are kidding,' he said. 'People worked hard on that exhibition and you trashed it. Tell me that you did not write that.'

'I did write it,' I said. I could not stop the slow laughing. 'Ha....'

On my second week in drug land, our shop had a visit from the directress of European stores. By then, I was in a completely catatonic state. I talked with her at length but could not remember most of the conversation hours later. In fact, I could barely keep my eyes open. I thought I might fall asleep whilst standing and drool on her beautiful Yves Saint Laurent shoes. I kept looking at her shoes to make sure that my spittle was not indeed on them. They were canvas, and I was sure that spit would stain. The thought made me want to laugh, but I could not. At that point, my face could no longer make different expressions. It had but one expression and that was *yeah, whatever.*

Most people noticed my condition. The UK area manager, who was *still* confused as to why I was *still* sick, told Simon, 'Poor Marlo could barely keep her eyes open when she was talking to the directress. I could see her struggling. She must have been in so much pain.'

Well, the pain was somewhere in the back of my thoughts. I knew it was there, but I didn't notice it too much. I was too preoccupied with trying not to drool all the time.

I realised that I could not function like this. I think we have all seen warnings on medicines that say 'Do not operate machinery whilst on this medication,' but I could barely operate my own body. The struggle became overwhelming.

I was supposed to stay on the drug for several weeks, but I decided to wean myself off on about the third week. I decided I would deal with the pain through mental strength, but that did not go well.

The pain got overwhelming again until a friend of mine gave me a small bag of marijuana. Pot was something that never really interested me. In high school, all the dumbest kids smoked it, so I didn't try it until I was well into my university years. I didn't like it when I tried it then, so I didn't really smoke it again.

The marijuana was the only thing that relieved the unbearable pain I was in. I didn't smoke it in the day, because I didn't feel comfortable coming to work high on an illegal drug. I would smoke it at night, and that was enough to get me through the night. I got a good night's sleep as well. The daytime was a different story.

Fatigue and pain continued to be problems for me over the next few months. It got to the point where William was taking off my shoes and socks at night. I would remove the rest of my clothes, and he would walk me to the shower, as I had slipped recently before. When my shower was over I would call him to help me get out.

'The carer is here,' he would joke.

'Soon you'll be wiping my ass,' I'd say.

'I wouldn't mind at all.'

One time I asked him, 'Will you mind changing my tampons too?'

'That's where I draw the line,' he said frowning.

Its one thing to have your husband help you wash and dress, but what happens to your self-esteem when colleagues try to help you? At work, one of my colleagues noticed that I was having a hard time taking off my trousers in the staff locker room. Without asking, she brought in a chair and told me to sit. She helped me change into my uniform.

I was initially a little sad and embarrassed and then I thought *Fuck it. All the best divas have someone help them dress.* It was a humbling gesture of kindness. As space in the locker room was already tight, the chair was in everyone's way, but no one moved it. She must have told them why it was there. I used it for the whole week, if not longer.

During this difficult time, my MS nurses referred me to a lovely occupational therapist called Pip. She was able to teach me ways of conserving energy, like placing kitchen utensils at waist level instead of above my head or way below. Not having to stretch up or way down conserves energy. She told me to use the lift instead of the stairs. She also advised me to take a twenty-minute nap during the day, which was very helpful.

I told Pip how I was getting so tired that I could barely hold on to the rail on the train in the mornings. Holding my arm up became exhausting and painful. The problem with MS (if you are not in a wheelchair or walking with a stick) is that most people cannot tell that there is something wrong with you. Because of this no one offers you a seat.

During my morning commute, I was dying inside. I felt like passing out on the floor every single morning. When I would get to Green Park tube station each morning, I would get back into my old habit of counting the steps. There are seventeen steps at the exit I used. I thought that if I didn't count them, then I wouldn't be able to get up them. *One, keep going. Two, keep going, three*, and so on.

With Pip's assistance, I was able to get approval for a government-assistance plan where a taxi would bring me to and from work for the price of my tube ticket.

But when the time came for the taxi to start picking me up, I cancelled the whole thing. In stubborn *Marlo* fashion, I referred to the film *Driving Miss Daisy*.

'I'm not going to be chauffeured around like an old woman,' I told William.

'What are you talking about? Everything is approved. Just take the taxis. You need to conserve energy!'

'No,' I said. 'I won't do it. I don't want it.'

As an alternative, I asked Simon if I could work one less hour a day. Instead of working nine hours, I wanted to work eight. He agreed and got approval from the company. Some days, I didn't need to work an hour less, so I would just stay. Other days, though, especially if I came in an hour later, it made a world of difference.

Because of my changed hours, I realised that some people began treating me differently. They would say little things like, 'I need an hour off in the morning. I have to make an appointment. Marlo does it.' I started to see that people in the workplace act differently to a disease when it is a chronic disease. It is one thing to get an illness, even get *very* sick, and then get better. Bosses can understand that scenario.

The problem with my scenario was that my bosses continued acting like they were wondering why I was still sick. So many times, one of them would say to me things like, 'Shouldn't you be feeling well by now?'

It became increasingly upsetting.

It all came to a head on a day that the European directress came for another visit. I had approached her regarding a colleague who was treating my staff members in an abusive manner. It was well known that this colleague had serious behaviour issues and often turned on people.

The directress's reaction to my complaint was shocking. I remember her words so well. She told me that the colleague in question had always been known as a rude woman with a poor attitude. She said that her poor attitude was worth enduring because the woman had helped the company a great deal and was organised and dedicated. She said people have different personalities and not everything is black and white.

'There is always grey area,' she went on to say. 'It is not easy for us to deal with a manager who is in your situation,' she said. 'It is not easy for the company and it is not easy for Simon, but we do it. We work around you, so you can work with us a little.'

My mouth dropped open. 'My *situation*?' I asked. 'I work harder than most people.'

'Harder than whom?' she asked and a full-blown argument ensued.

I left the room with a bright red face and the knowledge that I would never be given the opportunity to move up whilst she was in power. I knew I had the grounds for a lawsuit as well. Just months later, the Disability Discrimination Act 2005 would be passed in the UK, protecting the rights of people with MS.

I told Simon what had happened, and he insisted that she could not possibly have meant anything by it. He kept saying how much the directress liked me. He was not convincing, though. I quickly understood what was happening. His allegiance was with the company, so whether he was appalled or not, he couldn't show it. I couldn't really blame him.

I decided that day that I was going to resign. I just wasn't sure how soon. Everyone whom I told the story to said that I should get a solicitor. I didn't have the energy to. I was so overtired; I just wanted to leave and not have to deal with any of it.

Successes

§

My interest in work began to wane. As it did, my musical endeavours started to take on a new life. I performed my first solo gig in London. It was the first solo gig I had done in eighteen months. I wasn't nervous for it, as I was fed up about worrying that I could screw up. I remember thinking, *If Pete Doherty can be on stage drunk and drugged, then no one is going to care about a little brain disease making me wobbly.* The thought, *Fuck it, I still look good,* was becoming my permanent motto.

The first gig was successful. Lots of friends came and my performance was spot on. I played a second gig, which was another success. After my first two solo gigs, I contacted a charity I had heard of called Attitude is Everything, part of a bigger charity called Arts Online. Attitude's agenda was to make public music venues more accessible for people with disabilities. They put together gigs where four or five bands would play to raise money and awareness. Many of the bands had at least one member with a disability.

'If I have a disability,' I said to William one night, 'then I am going to make use out of it. I am going to make lemonade out of these lemons.'

'I agree,' he said, kissing my head. 'Start squeezing.'

So, I started embracing my MS as a disability and I began performing several gigs with Attitude is Everything. I played some fantastic venues, like Carling Academy in Islington. They also invited me to play in an international music festival called *In the City*, which took place in Manchester. It was an incredible experience.

William and I, accompanied by my three bandmates, trotted off to Manchester. We booked into the weirdest hotel we had ever been in: The Britannia. It looked like a ship that had been raised from the deepest ocean, where it must have sunk in the 1920s. It had a grand staircase that squeaked and shook as you climbed it. The hotel was dark and dismal. The air was thick. It was very spooky. Walking to our rooms, we saw that one room had been boarded up.

'What the hell is this?' William asked. 'It's like we are in a Stephen King novel. I don't think we are getting out of here alive!'

'We have no time to die, and it's like *Titanic* meets Stephen King,' I said. 'We have to get dressed and be on stage for the sound check in one hour!'

We did just that. We met many lovely people at that venue. Some were from Attitude is Everything, and others were fans, or friends. Many were in wheelchairs or with walking sticks. Some were blind, some were mentally ill. Many had diseases and conditions I had never heard of. People faced challenges that I hadn't thought of before. I began to realise how many challenges there are for those people with any disability, not just MS.

We played the gig to a packed crowd. The amount of adrenaline that went through me made me feel very high. As I belted out each song, I knew I was right where I was meant to be. I wasn't just meant to be on that stage. I was meant to be playing for a reason other than, 'Look at me.' My reason was now, 'Look at *us* (people with multiple sclerosis). Look what *we* can do. *We* are fucking unstoppable.'

On the train back to London the next day, I reflected on what a great night we had.

'Isn't it remarkable that I never would have met all these great people if I didn't have MS?' I whispered to William.

'You're making lemonade,' he answered, half asleep.

'I am learning so many things,' I said, closing my eyes and smiling.

෨

A great example of what I was learning occurred one day when I was waiting at a bus stop next to a girl in a wheelchair. The bus pulled in to the stop and left a huge gap between the curb and the bus. He opened the door and the girl told him he needed to pull up closer.

He looked put out by this and gave a little huff. He closed the door and tried to pull up closer. He came about two inches closer and opened the door again.

By this time an elderly man had walked up to the bus stop. The bus driver looked at the girl and huffed again! 'It's not close enough,' she told him. She was correct; it wasn't close enough. She could not wheel on and the bus driver obviously didn't care. It was shocking!

He left the door open as a protest that he wasn't going to try to get closer. In an instant, the elderly man and I locked eyes and nodded. Without words, we picked up the wheelchair with the girl in it and carried her onto the bus. I am sure that our combined anger gave us the strength, because neither of us was in any state to be doing what we did.

The whole scenario was a culmination of what I was learning about the difficulties for disabled people. I saw that our society had such a long way to go in understanding the needs of another human being. Getting MS had given me the opportunity to become more sensitive to other people's needs. It opened my eyes further and gave me more purpose. It gave my music more purpose. Now instead of just trying to 'make it' in music, my music could help open doors and raise awareness. I was pleased.

ಕಿ

As I continued to play more gigs, I also started to take better care of myself. Taking Lisa's advice, I started seeing a certified acupuncturist. I found her just down the road from our flat. She was incredible and I was lucky to find her. My sister had explained to me that a good acupuncturist will look at your tongue and feel your pulse. This acupuncturist did both. She also gave me Chinese herbs, which I found gave me energy. I still see her and I still take the herbs.

I also tried different vitamins, oils, lotions, and potions. Through trial and error, I found taking primrose oil to be greatly beneficial to me. I also started eating better. I ate more oily fish. I *tried* to eat less cheese. OK, I can't stop eating cheese every day! I love it!

I also started to rest when I felt tired. I was realising that like infections, *stress* was a trigger for my relapses. Every single time I had a relapse, I was either completely stressed out, had an infection, or both. I was now avoiding these two things fairly well.

As my body got stronger, so did my mind. I got more and more confident and realised that my decision to quit my job several months before now had to come to fruition.

৪১

The day I handed my resignation to Simon was unlike the previous time. This time, I felt almost nothing. I wrote that I was leaving for health-related reasons. That was not the whole truth, but I felt it was the neatest way to say goodbye. Simon was not surprised by the letter and accepted it without resistance.

I stayed on for three more months, as my contract required. It was also enough time for me to wrap things up there and hand over the department I had built, to the next empress or emperor. Because of my respect for my lovely staff, and because of my pride, I wanted to leave things in the best-possible order.

I was sad to leave Colin, whom I laughed with every single day. We worked so well together. However, we had become friends outside of work, so I knew I would still see him anyway.

Both of us became closer friends with Magdalara and Bruce and spent many an evening at their home chatting away about energy and spirits. I was discovering some of the things I wanted to learn about Magdalara from the beginning, part of my reason for not wanting to go back to the States.

🙰

In the summer of 2006, I was asked to play some summer festivals. This all came from contacts at Attitude is Everything. We played those gigs, which ended up being a prelude to the biggest show of all....

I received an email asking me to play Trafalgar Square for the mayor's annual Disability Rights Festival. I was asked how much money I would require to play the concert. Although I asked for a standard amount, it was a lot more than I have ever been paid to play. They agreed. It was a huge deal for me!

As my guitar player was on holiday, William agreed to play guitar for the concert. We needed a bass player, and I had the perfect idea for one. I got on the phone to Dave, our old bass player in New York.

'Dave, remember how you used to tell me about your fantasy?' I asked.

'Which one?' he asked, laughing.

I smiled deviously into the phone. 'The one where you carry your bass through JFK airport and tell pretty girls that you have a huge gig in London.'

'Yeah,' he answered, getting excited.

'I have a paid gig in Trafalgar Square with a projected audience of 2,000 people, if you would like to make that fantasy come true.'

'Oh my God!' he said. 'I am there.'

Weeks later, he was outside our flat with his bass and suitcase in hand.

'I can't believe I am here for a gig with you guys,' he said.

'I know.' I agreed. 'It's like old times, only bigger and better!'

I proceeded to tell him that we were due for a radio interview at a major London radio station in about three hours. This was all arranged through the festival promoters. They had asked me if I would be *willing* to do an interview! Dave was stunned by my news, and I whisked him away to the radio station.

'I can't believe any of this!' he kept saying, suffering from jetlag.

'It's great, isn't it?' I giggled and squeezed his arm.

We did a twenty-minute interview at the station and gave my CD to the DJ. He asked me questions about my music, multiple sclerosis, and the festival. He played two of my songs on the air as well. We had a great time. It was surreal for us! I was happy that my music was finally played on a London radio station, plus I was spreading the word about MS and disability in general.

Days later, after two nights of rehearsals with Dave, we were behind the set at Trafalgar Square. There were tents made up as dressing rooms. My dressing room was big and my name was written on a big paper taped to the wall.

'This is perfect for our little diva,' Dave commented.

'Yes,' William agreed, chuckling. 'This is definitely her style.'

When our turn came to play, we walked out onto the biggest stage we had ever played on. There were more people than we have ever played to! My heart raced with excitement! *Shall I say, 'Hello London!'? No, that is too corny!* I thought. I looked out and saw Colin and his partner in the audience. He had brought his sister as well. I was so happy to see them!

I looked at William and Dave and smiled wide.

'One, two, three, four,' and we were off! We performed every song like it was our last. I sang my heart out, completely crazed by adrenaline and the energy of the people and their applause and screams! I saw so many people with disabilities who were dancing, either on their feet or by wheeling their chairs. I felt great!

'When you hear the word *disability*,' I screamed out, 'Remember to focus on the *ability* part! You can do anything you put your mind to! Don't let anything or anyone stop you!'

The crowd cheered.

I finished the last song and said, 'I am so happy to play in my favourite city! Thank you!'

We walked off the stage like we were walking on clouds. William and Dave were ahead of me, and I somehow bumped into London Mayor Ken Livingstone. There were many photographers and press people who yelled at us to pose together while they clicked their cameras. Ken and I embraced and posed for hundreds of shots.

'Is London *really* your favourite city?' he asked me. 'You are from New York, aren't you?'

'Yes,' I answered. 'London *is* my favourite city.'

Going Back

In the six months that followed that great concert, I played smaller, but no less important, gigs and started to write more too. I played a gig at the famous One Hundred Club and donated the proceeds to the MS Society. I became more involved with the MS Society, and I saw it as an opportunity to learn and spread the word about multiple sclerosis.

I continued to use marijuana as my last resort whenever I was in excruciating pain that could not be helped by taking six Nurofen. I stopped *smoking* it, though, and began *eating* it instead. I did not want the harmful effects of marijuana smoke in my lungs. MS was enough of a problem without adding to it.

I tried to eat the marijuana plain, but that was, well, a bit disgusting. Instead, I began sprinkling some onto a well-known biscuit with a sponge cake base, coated with orange marmalade and chocolate. Let's pretend it's called, 'Faji cake'. I would then place another 'Faji cake' on top and bake it in the oven. I called it the 'Space Faji'.

I continued injecting my own ass, and established a lovely rapport with my team of MS nurses and doctors, a rapport that most people don't get to have with a medical team. I became involved with other studies they conducted, as I do to this day.

Whilst I was still employed at Yves Saint Laurent, I had been offered a job at my old company, Donna Karan. They knew I had MS and were quite accommodating.

The shop was in a historic townhouse that had five flights of stairs. They actually built me an office on an easily accessible floor, so that I did not have too many steps to walk up and down every day. I was astonished!

When the carpenter was building my office, he asked questions regarding where I wanted shelves, phone lines, and such. He measured the height of my desk by having me sit down and show him where I would like my elbows to rest. As I sat down, I asked him, 'Do you know why you are building this desk?'

His reply was something like, 'I don't know exactly why, but I know it's to help you.'

'I have multiple sclerosis,' I told him. 'Do you know what that is?'

He proceeded to tell me that he didn't know quite what it was, so I happily gave him a brief, but thorough, explanation. He commented that I looked so well that it didn't seem possible. I told him that looks can often be deceiving, especially in the world of MS.

'I'll let you get on with it,' I said finally. 'I just wanted you to know that you helped another human being today. I wanted to thank you.'

He gave a wide, genuine smile. 'You are very welcome,' he said, as I trotted away in my heels.

When I got back to the shop floor, I realised that there was something I needed to do. I felt some kind of closure was about to happen in my life, some sort of exhale. I was getting on with my life, but there was a place I needed to go to say a final goodbye to the *old Marlo*.

The next day was unusually clear and sunny. I left work a few hours early and headed for the train. My heart was racing with excitement as if I was going to see a friend I hadn't seen in ages. I could barely contain myself as I rode the train to the place where the ghost of *old Marlo* would be waiting: Canary Wharf.

I was going there for the first time since that day back in 2004. When I think of my MS, I think of it as having started its true life on that day when I first had blurry vision and felt the champagne bubbles in my head. I know from research that multiple sclerosis had probably been in my body long before that day, but psychologically, that day was still the beginning for me. That was the first *scare*: the first time my subconscious let me in on the changes that were occurring inside me.

When I emerged from the tube station at Canary Wharf, I almost didn't recognise it. It reminded me so much of Manhattan: something that hadn't even dawned on that fateful day. I had not seen it with such clarity.

I stood in awe as I looked to the right, observing all the restaurants, and then looked to the left, where the entrance to the mall was. I looked straight ahead towards the river.

'My God,' I whispered to myself, as my heart sank to my stomach.

I continued to look all around, recreating that terrible day in my mind. I remembered watching William walk towards the Citibank building to the right. I looked at the spot where he had told me to meet him; the spot that I almost didn't make it to.

I walked towards the mall where I had discovered the Boots the Chemist pharmacy. The mall entrance was actually on the lower level inside a building. I crossed a small street to get it. I did not remember that street being there, but I could see from the worn pavement that it was not new. I just hadn't seen it the first time. I had been too busy watching the raindrops tilt up and swing in front of my eyes.

I walked through the glass doors of the building. The first thing I saw was a bench. I swallowed a lump in my throat, as my eyes welled up with tears.

'There's where I left you, girl,' I whispered.

I saw everything transpire in front of me, as if it were a film. I remembered vividly how I had once stumbled through those doors and sat on that bench. I remembered how I thought I was having a stroke, or perhaps a heart attack. I remembered feeling confused and wanting the bubbles in my head to stop popping. Tears slowly fell down my face as I thought of how I had wondered if I would ever see William again.

I sat down on the bench and looked out the glass doors. I could see all the way across to the other side of Canary Wharf! I laughed to myself, stopping the flow of tears. I dug through my pockets for the tissues that I packed for this journey and wiped my face.

I could see *everything* that I could not see on that day. If I had been healthy that day, I *would have* been able to see William at his meeting spot, and I *would have* met him on time.

Whilst sitting there, I thought about how much had changed in my life since then. Here I was in the same exact spot as three years prior and yet I was not the same person at all. I had been on a roller coaster ride. Not just any old steel-framed smooth-riding roller coaster: no, one of the rickety wooden-framed, loud, wild, drop-you-200-feet kind.

I sighed. I was a changed person. Pain had changed me. Experience had changed me. Multiple sclerosis had changed me. I was not the girl I used to be.

I repeated those words in my head. *I'm not the girl I used to be.*

Suddenly, I smiled as if the sun was rising inside me. A warm feeling spread through every part of me as I continued thinking.

I am in fact, better than the girl I used to be. I am stronger and better in every way. Yes, I have become the awkward bitch, I thought. But the awkward bitch is like Supergirl's older sister, who the world is yet to know about; the wiser one with more experience. She still has the super powers, maybe more than Supergirl has. Although the awkward bitch bumps into things and wears an invisible helmet, she understands people better than Supergirl ever did!

I straightened my posture and put my tissues back in my pocket. *I would not change my life for anything. I have been through too much. I have learned too much. Now I know what I am made of. I am the fabulous, the gorgeous, the tenacious…. awkward bitch.*